A Guide to Ayurvedic Remedies

Dr Sonica Krishan, BAMS., ADNY., Ayurveda wellness guide and consultant, is an internationally recognized author and speaker. She is based in Chandigarh, India, and is a holistic living facilitator. Dr Sonica has authored five books on Ayurveda and natural health care, namely *Herbal Healers, Home Remedies, Healing through Ayurveda, Healing through Ayurveda Herbs in Your Kitchen Garden*, and *Healthy Living through Dosha Healing.* She has also worked as an editor for the Ayurveda section of *All Things Healing*, USA. Her articles have been published in *Hindustan Times, Times of India, Indian Express, Deccan Chronicle,* and *Dainik Bhaskar.*

A GUIDE TO AYURVEDIC REMEDIES

DR SONICA KRISHAN

hachette INDIA

First published in 2025 by Hachette India
(Registered name: Hachette Book Publishing India Pvt. Ltd)
An Hachette UK company
www.hachetteindia.com

1

ISBN 978-93-5731-611-8

Hachette Book Publishing India Pvt. Ltd
4th & 5th Floors, Corporate Centre,
Plot No. 94, Sector 44, Gurugram 122003, India

Typeset in Cambria 10.5/14.5
by InoSoft Systems, Noida

MIX
Paper | Supporting responsible forestry
FSC® C010615

Printed and bound in India
by Thomson Press India Ltd.

I dedicate my book to my affectionate family who bless and support my endeavour of holistic healthcare.

I dedicate my book to my affectionate family who bless and support my endeavour of holistic healthcare.

Contents

Introduction

Ayurveda is India's ancient healing wisdom that offers essential magnitude of preventive as well as curative potential for healthy existence and eminence. While the 5000-year-old Vedic astuteness inculcates all that is of prime importance to human life with infinite potential and holistic harmony, the intricately designed philosophy of Ayurveda about healing has a beautiful array of numerous positives for the health and well-being of an individual's body, mind and soul.

Science of Life

Ayurveda is the holistic ancient perception passed on by the learned sages of India, which has endowed our health and longevity with the virtues of natural wellness since time immemorial. The two meaningful words, *ayus* (life) and *veda* (knowledge or science) combine together to craft the word Ayurveda or the 'Science of Life'.

Ayurveda Treatment

Rightly regarded as *Sukha Chikitsa*, or blissful health management, Ayurveda logically means that which is the pure form of healing, wherein an individual may find complete relief from their ailment. At the same time, it ensures that, in the process, no other ailment crops up.

The Basics

Two key features are attributed to the entire science of Ayurveda:

1. *Swasthavritam* or natural lifestyle modification

This is the prophylactic approach to natural wellness in Ayurveda philosophy, which is manifested primarily by maintaining as well as sustaining holistic wellness. This is regarded as most imperative and desirable in Ayurveda discipline.

2. *Aaturvritam* or the curative aspect of Ayurveda therapy

Ayurveda, being a therapeutic discipline, has full potential to help a patient overcome the ailment from which he is suffering, using exclusively natural means of healing. Curing of a disease in Ayurveda is considered as secondary to harbouring of natural wellness.

Therefore, the Ayurvedic methodology to healthcare is extremely beneficial both in the preventive as well as curative arenas. Ayurveda believes that the human body is the sum total of *doshas,* or body humours, *dhatus*, or body tissues and *malas*, or body wastes.

This is evident from the Ayurveda adage – ***Dosha dhatu mala moolam hi shareeram.***

A natural balance of *doshas, dhatus* and *malas* is considered essential for the normal working of the body, as well as the mind.

The Five Elements in Ayurveda Philosophy

Our physical body is believed to be a natural amalgam of the five basic elements viz. sky or ether, air, fire, water and earth. This resonates with the theory of Ayurveda.

- *Aakasha* or ether (sky)
  This element is the empty space between the organs and cells.
- *Vata* or air
  This corresponds to all movements of the body.
  This is the implicit metabolic heat present within the body.
- *Jala* or water
  All the fluids flowing in the body like saliva, plasma, mucous, etc. correspond to the element of water.
- *Prithvi* or earth
  This manifests as our body substance.
- *Agni* or fire
  It governs the digestive system and metabolism.

The Three *Doshas*
An Introduction

The three *doshas*, or humours of the body, are the prime attributes that are significant for not only upholding the human body, but also in every little aspect that causes balance or imbalance within the body. *Vata* or air, *pitta* or fire and *kapha* or phlegm are entirely imbibed within the body. As long as the three *doshas* are present in their relative balanced states, an individual experiences natural wellness. However, when the three *doshas* become imbalanced, meaning either they are more or less than their normal limits, it causes disease.

Ayurveda Diet and Lifestyle Guidance

Diet and lifestyle are the two indispensable components of our everyday life. Ayurveda gives the complete responsibility of well-being, as well as the lack of it, to both these factors. Small alterations in everyday diet and lifestyle could remarkably improve your natural well-being!

Ayurveda Counsels Balance for Natural Well-Being

According to Ayurveda, the human body is composed of three fundamental elements: *doshas* (bodily humours), *dhatus* (tissues) and *malas* (waste products). This principle is reflected in the Ayurvedic adage: *Dosha dhatu mala moolam hi shareeram.* Maintaining a natural balance among these elements is considered essential for the proper functioning of both the body and mind.

Understanding *Dosha* Types – *Vata, Pitta* and *Kapha*

The human *prakriti* (innate personality) may broadly be categorized into three distinct types. These are the *vata* type, *pitta* type, and *kapha* type.

A person's *prakriti* comprises his/her physical attributes, mental characteristics and innate nature. *Prakriti,* or the basic constitution and temperament of an individual, is believed to remain more or less the same throughout his/her lifetime.

All these three – *dosha, dhatu and mala* – together make up the roots of the entire body. It has been said that an upsurge as well as deterioration of a tree depends mainly on the roots that make it; a similar experience is undergone by the human body.

The Ayurveda *Doshas* – *Vata, Pitta* and *Kapha*

Dosha, in Sanskrit, means 'that which vitiates.' Thus, *doshas* are the body humours that make up the body and yet they are very easy to vitiate.

Ayurveda believes that as and when the three *doshas* are in the state of natural equilibrium, these tend to sustain natural well-being. And on the contrary, when the *doshas* fall out of balance, then these are reason enough to make the body ailing.

The three *doshas* – *vata, pitta, and kapha* – govern various physiological and psychological functions in the body. They are dynamic in nature and are constantly influenced by our diet, lifestyle, emotions, and environment. When these *doshas* lose their natural equilibrium, they either increase or decrease, leading to imbalances that manifest as diseases.

Understanding the Three *Doshas*

1. ***Vata Dosha* (Air and Space Element)**

    - *Vata* is associated with movement, circulation and nervous system activity. It governs functions such as breathing, blinking, muscle contractions, nerve impulses and elimination.
    - Like the wind, *vata* is erratic, dry, light, cold, and mobile. It is responsible for eighty types of disorders, including joint pain, anxiety, constipation and dryness in the body.
    - *Vata* corresponds to the atmospheric air, influencing motion and flow in the body.

2. ***Pitta Dosha* (Fire and Water Element)**

    - *Pitta* regulates metabolism, digestion and transformation in the body. It governs body temperature, intelligence, appetite and the enzymatic processes necessary for energy production.

- *Pitta* is hot, sharp, oily, and intense, much like the sun. It is responsible for forty types of ailments, including acidity, inflammation, skin disorders and excessive anger.
- Just as the sun facilitates evaporation, *pitta* aids in absorption, assimilation, and digestion of food and experiences.

3. ***Kapha Dosha* (Earth and Water Element)**

- *Kapha* is responsible for structure, stability, lubrication, and immunity. It helps in tissue building, joint lubrication, and emotional calmness.
- *Kapha* is heavy, slow, cool, smooth, and moist, akin to the moon. It is responsible for twenty types of diseases, including congestion, weight gain, lethargy, and water retention.
- Just as the moon helps solidify and cool the environment, *kapha* nourishes, strengthens, and provides stability to the body.

Each individual has a unique balance of these three *doshas*, known as their *prakriti.* Maintaining harmony among them is key to health and well-being.

How To Use This Handbook

This handbook on Ayurveda for serious ailments is divided into twelve chapters.

The reader will find relevant details regarding signs/ symptoms of 'difficult to handle, but commonly experienced' diseases.

This book includes details regarding diet and lifestyle guidance.

Also, the reader will find appropriate information about herbs, home remedies, as well as classical Ayurvedic medicines that can be included in holistic and natural regimens.

Panchakarma

What is *Panchakarma*?

Ayurvedic *panchakarma* is a comprehensive detoxification and rejuvenation therapy based on ancient Indian medicine. '*Panchakarma*', as is evident from its name, means five methods of curing diseases.

1. *Vamana* – To cause vomiting
2. *Virechana* – To cause purgation
3. *Shirovirechana* or *Nasya* – Nasal errhine
4. *Asthapan vasti* – Enema to push medicines into the colon
5. *Anuvasan vasti* – Oil enema

These treatments aim to remove toxins, balance the *doshas*, as well as restore health. *Panchakarma* is customized for each individual patient and includes a series of steps, like oil massages and steam baths, to prepare the body for thorough detoxification. This all-encompassing approach not only addresses physical ailments but also fosters mental and spiritual well-being, making it a cornerstone of Ayurvedic healing.

How Can *Panchakarma* Help in Serious Diseases?

By boosting the body's natural healing processes, balancing the *doshas* and detoxifying the body, *Panchakarma* can help manage serious ailments. This comprehensive treatment is especially beneficial for long-term ailments like arthritis, neurological illnesses, autoimmune diseases and digestive disorders. The goal of these Ayurvedic treatments is to rid the body of deep-seated toxins and bring back balance, thus enhancing immunity and organ function in the end. *Panchakarma* largely cures illnesses by targeting their underlying causes, as opposed to simply treating the symptoms, and thus, it offers long-term benefits and improved overall health. It also promotes emotional stability and mental clarity, both of which are essential for handling serious diseases.

How *Panchakarma* Works

When you picture this paradigm, it becomes simple to understand the philosophy of *panchakarma*. There is a possibility that when a tree's branches and leaves are chopped off, they will eventually grow back. However, once a tree is uprooted, it cannot grow back. This is the *panchakarma* principle. According to Ayurvedic healing, on undergoing *panchakarma*, chances are few for a disease to recur, thanks to the five methods of body cleansing and restoration of health. *Panchakarma*, simply put, works on the principle of uprooting a disease from the body.

Why Ayurveda Recommends *Panchakarma*

There's a good reason that this cleansing mode has received so much attention. Ayurvedic medicine has two primary objectives:

1. To assist in preserving and retaining a person's health.
2. To eradicate a sick person's illness.

The five therapeutic modalities make it easy to accomplish both of these goals, which is why *panchakarma* has been valued for ages.

Philosophy of Ayurveda *Panchakarma*

A sickness develops if there is a shift in the body, whether it is seasonal or otherwise, that leads to an imbalance in the three fundamental body humours (*Doshas*), as identified by Ayurveda (*vata, pitta* and *kapha*). To eradicate the illness, the impaired *doshas* must be returned to their original state.

Different bodily parts become diseases due to disturbed *doshas.* It is easier to remove a sickness that is located in the alimentary canal, or *koshtha*, than it is when it appears inside bodily tissues, or *shakha*, as this requires more time and effort to treat. Furthermore, should the illness spread much farther, it tends to find its way into the *marmas,* or the deep-seated vital points. In this case, recovery takes considerably longer, and the disease may become rather incurable.

In Ayurveda, understanding the pathways and locations within the body is crucial for diagnosing and treating diseases. The terms *koshtha*, *shakha*, and *marma* are integral to this framework, each representing specific regions or aspects of the body's structure and function.

Koshtha

Definition: *Koshtha* refers to the body's internal cavities and hollow organs, primarily encompassing the gastrointestinal tract, including the stomach and intestines.

Significance: It is considered the central region where digestion and assimilation occur. The balance and movement of *doshas* (*vata, pitta, and kapha*) within the *koshtha* are vital for maintaining health. Imbalances here can lead to various gastrointestinal disorders.

Shakha

Definition: *Shakha* denotes the body's peripheral tissues, including muscles, fat, blood, and skin.

Significance: It represents the body's extremities and superficial tissues. When *doshas* become vitiated, they can migrate from the *koshtha* to the *shakha*, leading to diseases manifesting in these peripheral tissues. Understanding this movement is essential for effective treatment.

Marma

Definition: *Marma* points are vital anatomical locations where muscles, veins, ligaments, bones, and joints intersect. There are 107 identified *marma* points in the body.

Significance: These points are considered critical due to their association with essential life forces. Injury or trauma to *marma* points can lead to severe consequences, including pain, disability, or even death. They are central to various therapeutic practices, including *marma* therapy and Ayurvedic surgery.

Understanding these concepts is fundamental in Ayurveda, as they guide the diagnosis and treatment of diseases based on the movement and localization of *doshas* within the body's various compartments.

Ayurveda *Panchakarma* Techniques

Panchakarma techniques help in bringing the vititated *doshas* into the *koshtha*, where they can be more readily eliminated. The great teacher of Ayurveda, Charaka, emphasizes the necessity of oliation and fomentation of the body prior to executing these *Panchakarma*s. *Snehan* and *swedan karmas* are the names of these two techniques.

The use of a dry stick as an example helps to clarify why these are essential. A dry stick is more likely to break when bent, but not if it has been properly lubricated and heated previously. Likewise, with *snehan* and *swedan*, the *doshas* ensconced in bodily tissues become wet, lose their rigidity and stiffness and can be drawn into the *koshtha* (digestive tract) for discharge.

Panchakarma, derived from the Sanskrit terms *Pancha* (five) and *Karma* (actions), is a cornerstone of Ayurvedic medicine. It encompasses five primary therapeutic procedures designed to detoxify and rejuvenate the body, each targeting specific *doshas* (bodily humours) and ailments.

1. *Vamana* (Therapeutic Emesis)

Purpose: To expel excess *kapha dosha* (associated with mucus and phlegm) from the body.

Procedure: The treatment typically begins with preparatory procedures, including internal and external oleation (*snehana*) and fomentation (*swedana*), to loosen toxins. Following this, the patient consumes a medicated drink that induces controlled vomiting, thereby eliminating accumulated toxins from the upper gastrointestinal tract.

Indications: *Vamana* is particularly beneficial for conditions such as asthma, chronic allergies, bronchitis, and other respiratory issues linked to *kapha* imbalance.

2. *Virechana* (Therapeutic Purgation)

Purpose: To eliminate excess *pitta dosha* (associated with heat and bile) from the body.

Procedure: After preparatory treatments similar to those in *vamana*, the patient is administered herbal laxatives or purgatives to induce bowel movements. This process cleanses the small intestine and other *pitta*-dominated regions.

Indications: *Virechana* is effective for skin disorders, chronic fever, jaundice, and digestive issues arising from *pitta* imbalance.

3. *Nasya* (Nasal Administration)

Purpose: To purify and strengthen the head and neck regions by eliminating accumulated toxins.

Procedure: Medicated oils or herbal extracts are administered through the nostrils after a gentle massage and steam application to the head and face. This facilitates the removal of toxins from the nasal passages and sinuses.

Indications: *Nasya* is recommended for headaches, migraines, sinusitis, nasal congestion, and other head and neck disorders.

4. *Basti* (Therapeutic Enema)

Purpose: To balance *vata dosha* (associated with movement and dryness) by cleansing the colon.

Procedure: *Basti* involves the administration of medicated substances into the rectum. There are two primary types:

- ***Anuvasana Basti***: Uses medicated oils to lubricate and nourish.
- ***Niruha Basti***: Utilizes herbal decoctions to detoxify and cleanse.

Indications: *Basti* is beneficial for constipation, neurological disorders, arthritis, and other conditions related to *vata* imbalance.

5. *Raktamokshana* (Therapeutic Bloodletting)

Purpose: To purify the blood and alleviate disorders caused by blood impurities.

Procedure: This involves controlled removal of small quantities of blood using methods like leech therapy or venesection.

Indications: *Raktamokshana* is used for skin conditions, varicose veins, and other ailments stemming from blood impurities.

Note: *Panchakarma* treatments are highly individualized. Not all patients require all five procedures; the selection depends on the individual's constitution (*prakriti*), current doshic imbalances (*vikriti*), and specific health conditions. Due to the complexity and potency of these therapies, they should be administered under the supervision of a qualified Ayurvedic practitioner.

Understanding *Doshas* – *Vata*, *Pitta* and *Kapha* (Air, Fire and Phlegm)

Q. How can each *dosha* be balanced?

To Balance *Vata Dosha*:

Warm, moist and grounded foods, such as stews and soups, should be included in the diet on a regular basis. An optimum exercise schedule, soothing recreation and comforting tasks, like undertaking easy yoga poses and meditation, along with warm oil massages, like using sesame seed oil or mustard oil for relaxation and balance, should also be practised.

To Balance *Pitta Dosha*:

Eating more foods that are cold, hydrating and soothing, like melons and cucumber, and avoiding heat and strenuous activities are recommended. Relaxation and rejuvenation routines and massages with relaxing and cooling oils, like coconut oil, are also recommended.

To Balance *Kapha Dosha*:

It is necessary to undertake frequent and regular exercises and dynamic activities, avoid heavy and oily foods, as well as emphasize light, warm and spicy foods to boost metabolism. Conduct that encourages excitement and diversity is also recommended.

Q. How may a person with a particular *dosha* behave? What are their personality traits, attitude etc.?

***Vata* Type:** Individuals with a dominant *vata dosha* are often creative, lively and excited. As they, by and large, have rapidly fluctuating minds, they might also experience restlessness and weird habits. Often, these people could have trouble being consistent, and yet, their communication is brilliantly dynamic.

***Pitta* Type:** Individuals with a strong *pitta dosha* are often driven, determined and self-assured. They possess a sharp mind and are born leaders, but they could also be easily agitated, become impatient and possess a competitive spirit. They normally display a great sense of resolve and maintain a steady willpower.

***Kapha* Type:** Individuals with a dominant *kapha dosha* are composed and kind, and own a nurturing mental attitude. While they are dependable and patient, they might also experience sluggishness, inflexibility and reluctance to change. *Kapha* types commonly have calm and encouraging characteristics that act as a stabilizing influence.

Q. How can *doshas* intervene and co-exist (and how can they not)?

Doshas may co-exist or interfere depending on lifestyle choices and personal equilibrium. Each *dosha* supports the functions of the other in a balanced *dosha* state, which encourages health and harmony. On the other hand, abnormalities in one *dosha* can upset the balance and result in both mental and physical health problems. For instance, an overabundance of *kapha* can stifle *vata's* inherent vigour, whereas an excess of *vata* might dry out *pitta* and cause inflammation. To achieve optimal health and well-being, it is imperative to maintain a balance between the three *doshas*, enabling them to co-exist harmoniously.

Q. What are *doshas* and how are they categorized?

According to Ayurveda, an individual's physical and mental qualities are determined by the *dosha* that is foremost within them, which is a special mix of five elements (earth, water, fire, air and ether). Individuals are classified into three main *doshas*: *vata* (air and ether), *pitta* (fire) and *kapha* (earth and water). Each person's bodily type, mentality and health inclinations are determined by their unique combination of these *doshas*. This classification facilitates the creation of individualized wellness and treatment programmes that uphold equilibrium and well-being.

Q. Where do these *doshas* come from?

The five basic elements of nature – earth, water, fire, air, and ether, or the sky element – are the source of *doshas.* According to Ayurveda, these elements usually unite to generate the three *doshas*: *vata* (air and ether), *pitta* (fire) and *kapha* (earth and water). These *doshas* control a range of physiological and psychological processes in the body, impacting a person's behaviour, personality and general health. One's general state of health is determined by the balance of these *doshas,* and an imbalance might result in general health problems and serious diseases.

Q. Who came up with the theory of *doshas*?

The *dosha* concept originated in the 5,000-year-old Ayurvedic medicinal tradition. The *dosha* hypothesis is one of the core concepts of Ayurveda that are attributed to ancient philosophers and sages. Charaka and Sushruta, respectively, are notable authors of the fundamental texts, *Charaka Samhita* and *Sushruta Samhita.* These texts lay the groundwork for Ayurvedic knowledge by elaborating on the ideas of *doshas,* their functions and their implications for health.

Q. How does a *dosha* imbalance occur and how can it be balanced again?

Dosha imbalance is caused by various factors that disturb the natural equilibrium, such as eating bad food, stress, lack of sleep and environmental modifications. All *doshas* are susceptible to imbalance due to specific triggers:

1. ***Vata* Imbalance:** This is caused by unpredictable conduct, frequent travel, cold and dry weather and eating meals that are dry and chilly. The symptoms include dry skin, stomach issues, anxiety and insomnia.
2. ***Pitta* Imbalance:** This is generally brought about by intense heat, greasy or hot food, stress and intense physical activity. The symptoms are irritation, skin rashes, inflammation and acid reflux.
3. ***Kapha* Imbalance:** This particular *dosha* imbalance is brought on by overindulging, sedentary lifestyles, cold and damp weather and heavy and oily food consumption. The symptoms include depression, weight gain, congestion and lethargy.

To balance *doshas:*

Other than taking Ayurvedic medicines, balancing the three *doshas* also requires making dietary and lifestyle adjustments to offset the imbalance.

1. **Balancing *vata*** – Eating warm, nutritious meals, like soups and stews, that are moist, making and following a timetable and also engaging in calming activities, such as yoga and meditation, are recommended. Also, warm oil massage to relax and stabilize is considered beneficial.
2. **Balancing *pitta*** – Consuming hydrating and cooling foods like cucumbers and melons is good. Severe and intense heat conditions, exhausting exercise routines and consumption of hot or chilli-based meals should be avoided. Nevertheless, practising deep breathing, along with massages using soothing oils, like coconut oil, may also be beneficial.

3. **Balancing *kapha*** – Include brisk activities and frequent exercise. Warm, spicy and light foods aid metabolism. At the same time, avoiding oily or heavy foods, and engaging in activities that provide diversity and excitement also help.

In general terms, *dosha* imbalance is caused by various factors that disturb or increase/decrease the *doshas* from their natural equilibrium, such as consuming unsuitable foods repeatedly, undue stress and strain, lack of sleep, as well as environmental alterations. This makes the *doshas* susceptible to common and even serious diseases of the body and mind.

Furthermore, *panchakarma* and other Ayurvedic treatments, along with medicinal intervention, can aid the body's detoxification and *doshic* balance restoration for all the three *doshas* – *vata, pitta,* and *kapha.*

Disclaimer

The reader needs to understand that the treatments (medicine and remedies) mentioned in this book are mainly for reference purposes. You must discuss with your Ayurvedic doctor or *Vaidya* as the required dosage may vary according to your age and physical condition.

However, as per Ayurvedic herb recommendations, for an adult, the dosage is mentioned in general scenario, while the dose would be half for children. Generally:

1. Fresh juice extracted by pounding or crushing the herb is 10–20 ml, to be taken twice a day.
2. Dosage for powders is 3–5 grams. It is better that these be taken along with some warm water.
3. Recommended dosage of decoction (*kadha*) prepared from the herb is generally 50–100 ml, which may be taken twice a day.
4. *Asav/Arisht*: 25–30 ml, mixed in an equal quantity of water, to be taken twice a day, after meals.

5. Ghee/*Ghritam* medicinal preparations: 5–10 ml, along with warm water.
6. *Avleha*: 6–15 grams, once or twice a day.
7. Tablets (may be referred to as *vatti* or *gulika*): 1–2 tabs, twice a day.
8. *Churan* (Medicinal powder): 5–10 grams, twice a day, along with warm water.
9. Also, it needs to be understood that, as classical Ayurvedic medicines would generally contain purified metals or some herbo-minerals, they must be strictly decided by the vaidya in charge.
10. For the 12 diseases that are cited in the book, it needs to be ascertained that although the required *panchakarma* therapies have been mentioned, yet the remaining *panchakarma* therapies (if needed) may be decided by the treating Ayurvedic physician on a case-to-case basis.

Chapter 1

DIABETES

Disease Introduction

Diabetes mellitus, known as *madhumeha* in Ayurveda, is a chronic and serious disease wherein there is defective metabolism. In this particular disease, the patient experiences persistent and recurrent passing of urine in large quantities. Diabetes patients generally present as insulin-dependent and non-insulin-dependent.

In Ayurveda, *madhumeha* is a condition that closely resembles diabetes mellitus. It is classified under *prameha*, a group of urinary disorders, and is considered a *mahagada* – a severe and chronic disease. This severity is attributed to the significant impairment of *vyadhikshamatva* (immunity), which is linked to an individual's *bala* (strength). In *madhumeha*, there is a depletion of *ojas* – vital essence responsible for immunity and overall vitality – leading to *ojas kshaya* (loss of *ojas*). According to Ayurvedic texts, *ojas* is the supreme essence of all the body's tissues (*dhatus*) and is crucial for sustaining life. Therefore, the loss of *ojas* in *madhumeha* adversely affects the entire immune system.

Ayurvedic Understanding of the Disease

Prakrashtm mehti yasmin roge sa prameha

Factors, related to food and daily or seasonal regimen, that contribute to *madhumeha* include:

a. Overindulging in food without digesting previously consumed food
b. consuming new grains excessively
c. High-calorie diet
d. *Guru, snighdha, sheeta, manda, shlakshna, sandra, sthira* and *pichchila guna ahara* (mostly, heavy, slimy, cold foods)
e. Excessive jaggery-based or sweetened food item
f. Excessive *dahi* (curd intake)
g. Sleeping during the day
h. Laziness
i. Not undergoing the detoxification processes.

These essential factors of *ahara* and *vihara* (diet and lifestyle), which are regarded as *madhumeha nidana*, are dominant in the disease of diabetes. A person's tissue microenvironment is affected by inadequate as well as excessive nutrition, which compromises both the structure and function of the body and lays the ground for the disease.

The disease in which there is repeated urine output, in large quantities is referred to as *prameha* (diabetes) in Ayurveda.

Ayurvedic text mentions that the urine of a diabetic person is sweet, and thus this disease is mentioned as *madhumeha*, wherein *madhu* means honey. Although there is mention of 20 types of *prameha rogas*, or urinary diseases, it is notable that when *pramehas* become chronic and give way to a serious disease, they cause *madhumeha* or Diabetes Mellitus.

Twenty types of *prameha* have been mentioned. Of these,

1. Four types are considered incurable. These are believed to be formed mainly due to the vitiation of *vata dosha*, or the air body humour.
2. Six types are believed to be formed by the vitiation of *pitta dosha*, or the fire body humour. These are considered difficult to cure.
3. Ten types of diabetes, which develop due to the vitiation of *kapha dosha*, or phlegm body humour, are believed to be curable.

Signs and Symptoms:

1. The frequency of urination, in large amount and with low specific gravity, increases. This is generally termed as Polyuria.
2. Increased thirst.
3. Burning sensation in the palms and soles.
4. Body weakness and lethargy.
5. Pain in calf muscles is a common feature.
6. Diabetic degeneration.
7. Sleep disturbance.
8. Late healing or non-healing of wounds.
9. Muscle wasting.
10. Itching all over the body.
11. Blood sugar level remains above 120 mg (fasting) and above 180 mg (P.P.)

In Ayurveda, *madhumeha* is one of the twenty types of *prameha* (urinary disorders) mentioned in nearly all classical texts, and it closely resembles diabetes mellitus in modern medicine. If *prameha* is not properly managed, it can gradually develop into *madhumeha*, a more severe condition.

Acharya Sushruta, in *Chikitsa Sthana*, categorizes *prameha* into two types:

1. *Apathya Nimittaja Prameha* – Acquired diabetes, caused by an unhealthy lifestyle and diet.
2. *Sahaja Prameha* – Hereditary diabetes, present from birth due to genetic factors.

According to Acharya Charaka in the *Charaka Samhita*, *madhumeha* is classified as a *mahagada* or *maharoga*, meaning it is a chronic and severe disease with serious health consequences.

The early warning signs (prodromal symptoms) of *prameha* include:

- Excessive coating (*mala*) on the tongue, palate, and teeth
- Burning sensation in the hands and feet
- Oily or greasy skin and body
- Excessive thirst
- A persistent sweet taste in the mouth

Proper management through diet, lifestyle changes, and Ayurvedic treatments is crucial to prevent the progression from *prameha* to *madhumeha*.

Diet and Lifestyle Management Tips:

- It is necessary to choose the right grains and food options for diabetic patients.

- Avoid sweets and sweet/sugary foods.
- Restrict the intake of rice, maize, sweet potatoes, potatoes, sweetened fruits and fruit juices; hard drinks, non-vegetarian foods, high fat curds and highly spiced and fried foods.
- Use utensils made from the wood of Vijaysaar tree for eating and drinking.
- Avoid sleeping during the day.
- Do some light exercises and take long walks in fresh air for at least 2–3 kilometres.
- Practise pranayama, or the deep breathing techniques, every day.
- Perform yogic exercises, like *Surya Namaskar*, *Ardha Matsyasana*, *Bhujang Asana*, *Dhanur Asana*, *Mayur Asana* etc., regularly.
- Try to avoid physical injuries as much as possible.
- Monitor your blood-sugar level occasionally.

Recommended Home Remedies

- Drink about 10 to 20 ml of fresh juice of amla (Indian gooseberry) on empty stomach, once or twice daily.
- Soak 1 teaspoon fenugreek seeds (*methi dana*), overnight, in a glass of water. Drink this water on empty stomach in the morning.
- *Bilva* or *bael* (Aegle marmelos) can help decrease blood sugar levels and control excessive urination. It is beneficial to drink the juice extracted from the leaves of *bael* on empty stomach. Prepare this by crushing or pounding fresh leaves of *bael*. Consume it in doses of 2 teaspoons once or twice a day.

- Chapattis prepared from roasted *jau* (barley) is recommended. Alternatively, chapattis may be prepared using five parts of *jau* flour mixed into 1 part of *chana* or gram flour.
- Consume one teaspoon of the powder prepared by crushing the dried seeds of *jamun* (*Syzygium cumini*), twice a day preferably, with warm water.
- Chew 3 to 5 fresh leaflets of *neem* (*Azadirachta indica*) first thing in the morning. Alternatively, the *neem* leaves may be crushed and made into a paste. This may be taken in doses of one teaspoon along with some warm water.
- Drink 10 to 20 ml of *karela* (bitter gourd) juice in the morning; also, include the vegetable in your diet.
- Pound some fresh mango laves (approx. 1 teaspoon) and make it into a juice. Mix it in an equal quantity of *karela* juice and drink the mixture on empty stomach. This is beneficial in the initial stages of diabetes.
- Mix some turmeric powder or *haldi* (preferably raw turmeric) with an equal quantity of dried *amla* powder. Take one teaspoon once or twice a day.

Other Herbs that Help

- *Brahmi* (Centella asiatica)
- Coconut (Cocos nucifera) flowers
- Fresh mango leaves
- Paste of *palash* flowers (Butea monosperma)
- *Tulsi* leaves (holy basil)
- Groundnut flour

The Ayurvedic classics provide a thorough understanding of the patho-physiology of diabetes mellitus, which is characterized by fire (*agni*) depletion, disruptions in the metabolism of fat (*meda*) and a weakened immune system (*ojas*). Along with a modified diet and lifestyle, the primary treatment approaches for this disease appear to be the promotion of *agni* and *ojas*, and the rectification of *meda*. Acharya Charaka also refers to *madhumeha* as *ojomeha* in *Chikitsa Sthana* within the context of *ojas*. Ayurveda does not view diabetes mellitus as a condition that can be cured by diet or medication alone. It is mentioned in *Charaka Samhita* that diabetes mellitus is a *yapya* disease, meaning one that is difficult or impossible to cure.

Classical Ayurvedic Drugs

- *Chander prabha vatti*
- *Shilajitvaadi vatti*
- *Agnitundi vatti*
- *Shudh shilajtu*
- *Dhanvantara ghrita*
- *Vasant kusumakar rasa*
- *Brihat bangeshwar rasa*
- *Mal sindoor*
- *Swarna rajbangeshwar rasa*
- *Banga bhasm*
- *Dashmoolarishta*
- *Madhumehari yog*
- *Balarishta*
- *Tribanga bhasm*
- *Arogyavardhani gutika*
- *Triushanaadi lauh*
- *Abhyaadi modak*
- *Yashad bhasm*

- *Trivang bhasm*
- *Satv giloy*
- *Jatiphal vatti*
- *Narsimha churan*

Panchakarma Therapies

Diabetes frequently causes an imbalance of the *kapha dosha,* and the *panchakarma* therapy of *vamana* (therapeutic emesis) assists in removing the same. Also, another *panchakarma*, i.e. *virechana* (purgation therapy), helps to improve digestion and metabolism by eliminating excess *pitta dosha* and toxins from the intestines and liver. Moreover, *basti* therapies (medicated herbal enemas) help to regulate *vata dosha,* facilitate better bowel motions, strengthen pancreatic function and enhance the health of the nervous system. Other therapies that are advised are *udvartana* (herbal powder massage) and *shirodhara* (oil dripping therapy).

> According to Ayurveda, the etiological factors for *madhumeha* include a sedentary lifestyle, excessive consumption of heavy, unctuous, and saline-tasting foods, new cereals and large quantities of fresh wine, as well as not engaging in any physical or mental exercise, or body-cleansing procedures.

Udvartana is a dry-powder massage, recommended as an external treatment to improve fat metabolism, increase blood flow and control obesity, all of which are frequently linked to diabetes. As *udvartana* is extremely dry, it helps diabetics lose body fat and nullifies the aggravated *kapha.* On the other hand, *shirodhara* (oil dripping therapy) aids in balancing the mind and body, thereby reducing stress, which is essential in diabetes disease management.

Other causes of diabetes, as mentioned in Ayurveda, are:

- ***Asyasukham:*** Cozy and comfortable sitting for long durations (sedentary lifestyle, lack of exercise and physical inactivity).
- ***Svapnasukham:*** Excessive sleeping and luxuries of overindulging in sleep.
- ***Kaphakrut Cha Sarvam:*** Diets and lifestyle that elevate the *kapha dosha*.
- ***Etiological factors:*** *Sahaja* (inherited factor); *chinta* (stress); *shoka* (grief); *bhaya* (fear); *deergharoga* (long-term disease) and *alasya* (sedentary living).

Diabetic individuals are advised to engage in strenuous exercise. This helps the body to use up the accumulated fat and break down glucose in the right way. These techniques can be modified based on the time (*kala*) and the habitat (*desha*). Among the challenging yet beneficial activities that Sushruta recommends are:

- Workouts (*vyayama*)
- Fighting (*niyudidha*)
- Games (*kreeda*)
- The ability to ride an elephant, horse, cart, walk and so on (*gajacharya, turagacharya, rathacharya* and *padacharya*)

Some Ayurvedic facts about Diabetes:

1. Indians have known about diabetes mellitus since the Vedic era, when it was referred to as *asrava* (*prameha*).

They were handling this issue quite skilfully. Ayurveda categorizes *prameha* into three main types: 1. *kapha* type (split into 10 categories); 2. *pitta* type (split into six types); and 3. *vata* type (four varieties in all). The primary contributing factors are considered to be sedentary lifestyle, excessive consumption of sugary, non-vegetarian foods and dairy products, jaggery (preparations made from cane sugar) and large, overindulgent meals. The *vataja pramehas* of Ayurveda mention that diabetes is treatable if one exercises caution in food practices, exercise and medication. Herbal treatments for diabetes include using *gudmar* (Gymnema sylvestre), *asana* (Pterocarpus marsupium), *khadir* (Acacia catechu), *lodhra* (Symplocos racemosa), *guduchi* (Tinospora cordifolia) and *jambu* (Syzygium cumini).

2. The entire spectrum of diabetes, including its etiology, pre-clinical and clinical aspects and consequences, as well as its stage-by-stage management, is eloquently portrayed in Ayurveda. It is difficult for someone who is focussed on diabetes prevention to overlook the pre-clinical description of *prameha*, or *madhumeha*, as diabetes management is described in Ayurveda. Patients who are heavy and well-built should follow Acharya Charaka's advice and adopt samsodhana *chikitsa*; while those who are underweight and weak should receive *bruhana* therapy. Sushruta says that, while fat people should be treated with apatarpana methods (*vyayama* and *shodhana*), *krusha pramehi* should be treated with *santarpana chikitsa* (processed diet and drink). *Chikitsa*, or treatment, is composed of *ausadhi* (medication),

vihara (exercise and yoga) and *ahara* (food). Since it is clear that *prameha* is dominated by *kapha dosha* and that dushya *meda* is similar in character. Ayurveda suggests the use of drugs with the *rasa* qualities of *tikta* (bitter), *katu* (pungent) and *kashaya* (astringent) for the treatment of *prameha*. Sushruta explicitly prescribes the infusion of medications with *shilajit* to treat *madhumeha*.

3. The first documented history of diabetes dates back to 200 BC and may be found in the ancient texts from Egypt, Greece, China and India. Diabetes is named after the urine of a person with the sweet taste of honey. The elaborate description of diabetes and its management under a condition diagnosed as *madhumeha* and *prameha* can be found in ancient Ayurvedic scripts related to medicine and surgery, such as in the *Charaka Samhita*, *Sushruta Samhita* and *Vagabhatta*.
4. Since *madhu* and mellitus both signify honey, the terms *madhumeha* and diabetes mellitus are thus synonymous. Ayurveda employs a mix of nutritional supplements, lifestyle modifications and therapies to manage and even reverse diabetes. The Ayurvedic approach to diabetes treatment involves certain dietary restrictions and suggestions, including *shodhana* (Ayurvedic detoxification, like *panchakarma*), yoga poses and Ayurvedic herbal medicines. As for preventing *madhumeha*, *ahara chikitsa* (diet therapy) is suggested. All the classical texts strongly recommend *nidana parivarjana*. Therefore, the patient is advised to follow a diet (*ahara*) that does not increase body weight and is contrary to the etiological factors of *prameha*/

madhumeha. Since diabetes is understood to be a disease of altered lifestyle and defective *agni*, nutrition and bio-purifying practices should receive more attention. The diabetic individual, or pramehi, should take yava, as a general diet, according to Charaka. Along with this, *vihara* (workout) is recommended. Another major contributing factor to the etiology and pathogenesis of *prameha/madhumeha* is excessive daytime and oversleeping, combined with a lack of exercise. According to Sushruta, this particular disease should be approached by frequent physical exercise, wrestling, real sports, riding horses or elephants, taking long walks, travelling or brisk walks, practising archery, throwing javelins and other physical activities.

5. Regular exercise (*vyayama*), as part of the *dinacharya* (daily regimen), with characteristics of *Balardha Yoga* (exercise up to half strength) may help control diabetes mellitus. Patients with type 2 diabetes mellitus are advised, in their initial care, to focus on diet, physical activity and weight loss. Adhering to the ashtvidha *ahara* visheshayatan and dwadasha ashana vichara (the eight and 12 rules for diet intake) can be a powerful preventive measure against the risk of diabetes mellitus as Ayurveda views sedentary lifestyle (*asyasukham*) and a high-calorie diet (*guda vaikritam*) as major contributing factors to *madhumeha*. Diabetes mellitus has been linked to the ailment known as *prameha*, which is caused by *mutravaha srotasa*, with the dominance of *kapha*. *Madhumeha* is a subtype of *prameha* that falls under the *vataja* type. It is characterized by the flow of urine that is sweet, like honey, and by the sweetness

of the entire body. *Madhumeha* can be avoided by practising preventative techniques, as prescribed in Ayurveda, including *dincharya*, *ritucharya*, and *aharavidhi* in conjunction with therapeutic techniques.

KEY TAKEAWAYS

- *Madhumeha* (diabetes) is considered a severe disorder in Ayurveda because it depletes *ojas*, the vital essence responsible for immunity and overall well-being, leading to weakened immunity and chronic health issues.
- If *prameha* (urinary disorders) is not properly managed, it can progress into *madhumeha* (diabetes), a severe and chronic condition. Ayurveda emphasizes early detection, lifestyle modifications, and dietary changes to prevent this progression and maintain overall health.
- Managing diabetes with Ayurveda involves a balanced diet, regular exercise, mindful lifestyle choices, and holistic practices like yoga and pranayama. Avoiding sugary and high-carb foods, staying active, using natural remedies like Vijaysaar wood, and monitoring blood sugar levels can help maintain overall health and prevent complications.
- Ayurveda views diabetes (*madhumeha*) as a complex, long-term condition linked to weakened digestion (*agni*), fat metabolism (*meda*), and immunity (*ojas*). Management focuses on boosting *agni* and *ojas* while correcting *meda*, rather than relying solely on diet or medication. According to *Charaka Samhita*, diabetes is a *yapya* disease, meaning it requires continuous management rather than a complete cure.

- Ayurveda has recognized diabetes (*prameha*) since the Vedic era and classifies it into *kapha*, *pitta*, and *vata* types. Lifestyle choices, diet, and sedentary habits are key contributors. However, *vataja prameha* suggests that diabetes can be managed with proper diet, exercise, and medication. Traditional Ayurvedic herbs like *gudmar*, *asana*, *khadir*, *lodhra*, *guduchi*, and *jambu* are used for treatment.
- The first recorded history of diabetes dates back to 200 BC, with references in ancient Egyptian, Greek, Chinese and Indian texts. In Ayurveda, diabetes is described as *madhumeha* or *prameha*, with detailed management guidelines found in classical texts like the *Charaka Samhita*, *Sushruta Samhita* and *Vagabhatta*.

Chapter 2

ASTHMA

Ayurvedic Name: ***Tamak Shwas***

Disease Introduction

Ayurveda specifies that when *vayu* (air body humour) moves upwards, reaches the *srotas,* or minute channels of the body, and constricts the neck and head region, it aggravates *kapha* or phlegm, which produces a wheezing sound from the throat. This condition is tormenting for the patient who experiences acute spasm, with frequent bouts of dry cough. It continues until the phlegm is expelled. Only then, the sufferer finds temporary relief.

Ayurvedic Understanding of the Disease

In Ayurveda, asthma is believed to originate from affliction of the stomach and gastro-intestinal tract. This can be confirmed from the fact that in the initial stages of the disease, the patient shows signs of indigestion accompanied by diarrhoea or constipation. Though, the main affected organ is the

The clinical manifestation of bronchial asthma bears a strong resemblance to *tamaka shwasa* in Ayurvedic medicine. *Tamaka shwasa* literally translates to "burying into darkness due to shortness of breath." *Tamaka* means "darkness" and *shwas* means "shortness of breath." Prolonged exposure to *hetu* (causative factors), according to Ayurveda, impairs the actions of the *prana vayu,* which first damages the lungs structurally and then changes the lungs' natural elasticity and smoothness into hardness and roughness. Along with *sakashta* and *sashabda shwas,* this causes a rise in mucous secretions, which eventually dry out owing to *ruksha guna* (roughness) of *vata* and accumulates in the bronchial passages, making breathing harder. This is explained as a *yapya vyadhi* in Ayurveda.

lung. Constant pressure on the lungs even affects the heart. Therefore, while treating the disease, proper attention is given to the working of the stomach, bowels, lungs, nasal region and the heart (in chronic cases).

Bronchial asthma, known in Ayurveda as *tamaka shwasa,* is thoroughly detailaed in the *Charaka Samhita.* There is mention of various methods of treating *shwasa roga* (asthma). The ancient Ayurvedic books include extensive documentation on asthma. The Sanskrit term for asthma is *shwasa roga.* While *shwasa* means breathing in and out, *roga* means disease. There are five different kinds of asthma, according to *Charaka Samhita: maha shvasa, urdhva shvasa, chinna shvasa, tamaka shvasa* and *ksudra shvasa.* While the first three kinds are incurable. *tamaka shvasa* is considered to be difficult to cure, and yet can be controlled. However, the final one is treatable. Poly-herbal combinations are considered to be among the most widely recognized, secure and successful forms of treatment for asthma.

Signs and Symptoms

- Difficulty in breathing, and a feeling of constriction and tightening around the chest
- A wheezing sound when breath is expelled
- A feeling of suffocation during recurrent attacks
- There is fighting for the breath, prolonged expiration and short and gasping inspiration
- Bouts of cough along with tenacious and mucoid sputum
- In chronic cases, the face turns pale and the body becomes emaciated.
- Rhonchi sounds from the chest
- Laboratory findings show increased number of eosinophils.

A thorough explanation of *shwasa* and its five variants can be found in the seventeenth chapter of the *Charaka Samhita*. A methodical description of the pathogenesis, prodromal symptoms, clinical presentations, etiology, along with management of *shwasa* is provided. *Charaka Samhita* states that there are numerous fatal illnesses. However, none of these conditions are as fatal as asthma and hiccups. Both of these diseases are believed to originate at the site of *pitta* (in the stomach) and are caused by the simultaneous aggravation of *kapha* and *vata doshas. Charaka Samhita* also mentions that this particular disease has a negative impact on every tissue component, including the heart region.

Diet and Lifestyle Management Tips

- Light, warm to hot and easily digestible food is recommended. Sour foods, curd, butter milk, cold drinks and fried foods must be avoided.

- Dinner should especially be taken very light and early.
- Use hot water for drinking as well as for bathing.
- Banana, guava, pineapple and oranges are some fruit restrictions.
- During asthmatic attacks, small and frequent sips of hot water or ginger tea are good.
- Avoid smoking and consumption of alcohol.
- Pranayamas or deep breathing exercises are beneficial.
- Morning walks, preferably in the sun, helps.
- Avoid cold and damp environmental conditions.
- Avoid fumes, dust, polluted air and smoke.
- Maintain a relaxed mental attitude and keep away from mental stress and strain.

> *Vata* is dry, cold, rough and movable, while *kapha* is cold, heavy, slimy and unctuous. As *kledaka kapha* builds up, it travels to the lungs. When the two combine in the lungs, the mucous thickens and becomes gluey, sticking to the bronchial walls and constricting the bronchial tubes, which can result in asthma attacks or dyspnoea. As *Charaka Samhita* states, in case the *vata dosha,* which is mainly associated with *kapha*, obstructs the channels and circulates throughout the body, this aggravated *vata dosha* causes *shwasa roga* since it is blocked. "Moving in reverse encompasses the channels of vital breath, faultily affects the neck and head region and stimulates phlegm or the *kapha dosha,*" is how the scripture characterizes retrograde *vata*.

Recommended Home Remedies

1. It is crucial to be aware of the allergens that trigger the symptoms, and thus, to avoid the same.
2. A teaspoon of turmeric powder, taken twice a day, along with hot water, proves beneficial.

3. A decoction prepared from boiling equal parts of ginger, holy basil and black pepper, mixed with half a teaspoon of honey, is to be taken. Take this warm, in a dose of 20 ml, twice a day.
4. A powder prepared from dried and pounded herbs (black pepper, ginger and *pipali*) is to be taken along with warm or hot water. This helps to relieve the bronchial spasm.
5. A teaspoon of honey, with a few drops of ginger juice added to it, is to be taken on empty stomach in the morning.
6. Apply or massage some *til taila* (sesame seed oil) on the chest, followed by hot fomentation.
7. In bronchial asthma, when phlegm remains stuck in the bronchioles, *ajwain* helps to reduce the excessive production of phlegm. For this purpose, you could either take it in the form of powder, twice daily, or even make a decoction with the herb and take it warm.
8. The smoke that results from burning *hing* (asafoetida) can be inhaled for relief from spasms of bronchial asthma.
9. Being antiseptic in nature and a destroyer of phlegm, betel is used for treating bronchial asthma. As a home remedy, try mixing some juice extracted from betel leaf (5–10 ml approx.) with freshly ground basil, mint and ginger. Add 4–5 pounded pepper to the paste. Half a teaspoon of this preparation can be taken twice, along with some honey.
10. Mint is also recommended as a home cure for asthma due to its property of extracting and decreasing phlegm. Extract some juice by crushing fresh mint leaves. Add

to this an equal quantity of ginger juice. 5–10 ml of the mixture can be taken twice a day, along with honey.

11. *Tulsi* also contains specific anti-asthmatic properties. Fresh juice produced by pounding some *tulsi* leaves is to be taken twice. To this, you could add a few drops of ginger and some honey. This also helps to build resistance against the disease.
12. Camphor helps to loosen the phlegm and make the expectoration easy. You could massage the throat externally with camphor added to mustard oil. This also helps to relieve sore throat.
13. Steam inhalation with *ajwain* water is beneficial.

Other Herbs that Help

- Cardamom (Elettaria cardamomum)
- *Kantkari* (Solanum xanthocarpum)
- Clove (Syzygium aromaticum)
- Garlic
- Black pepper
- Grapes (Vitis vinefera)
- Mint (Mentha spicata)
- *Adusa* (Adhatoda vasica)
- *Tulsi* (Ocimum sanctum)
- Asafoetida (Ferula foetida)
- Mulethi (Glycyrrhiza glabra)

Classical Ayurvedic Drugs

- *Swas kuthar rasa*
- *Swas kas chintamani rasa*
- *Swas kuthar rasa*
- *Sitopladi Cchuran*

- *Dashmoolarist*
- *Kanakasava*
- *Chyavanprash avleha*
- *Agastya rasayan*
- *Vasa churan*
- *Shukti bhasm*
- *Shankh bhasm*
- *Suvarna – pushpasuga rasa*
- *Trikuti churan*
- *Antamool ghan vatti*

Panchakarma

Vaman and *virechana*, the two *panchakarma* remedies, are useful Ayurvedic treatments for asthma. Removing excess *kapha* from the respiratory tract by *vaman* (therapeutic emesis) helps clear congestion and mucous. Purgation therapy, or *virechana*, increases metabolism, balances the vitiated *pitta dosha* and detoxifies the body. These treatments seek to improve lung function and reduce asthma symptoms organically, in conjunction with a customized diet and lifestyle adjustments.

Asthma is treated in Ayurveda by identifying the *doshic* imbalance. In order to fully anticipate the healing process, the patient must be willing to alter their food and way of life, look for emotional and mental triggers for their illness, remove the cause, boost immunity, develop disease resistance and lead a peaceful life. Although the primary method of treating Asthma is *panchakarma*, which removes impurities and cleanses the body, palliative care may be necessary for many patients who lack the energy or health to perform the processes of *panchakarma*.

Some Ayurvedic facts about Asthma:

1. *Charaka Samhita* and *Ashtanga Hrdayam* both describe asthma in comparable ways. Pointing out that *kapha* vitiates the channels of *prana* (breathing), *udaka* (water) and *anna* (food), which are located in the chest, and creates *shwasa*, which emerges from the stomach, obstructing *vata*'s movement, spreading in all directions. 'Sensation of pain in the area of the heart and flanks, upward movement of *prana* (respiration), occasional flatulence, as well as splitting pain in the temples' are the prodromal symptoms of the disease of asthma. Also, Ayurveda believes that *tamaka* shwas can be associated with the clinical demonstration of bronchial asthma. According to *Shodhana Chikitsa, Shamana Aushadhis* and *Sthanika Chikitsa*, Ayurvedic treatment is advised for managing this disease. Moreover, *Nidana Parivarjana* implies stringent instructions to prevent triggering the disease's internal pathology.
2. Etiological factors that are similar to those mentioned from a modern perspective are described in the *Charaka Samhita*. Majority of the etiological causes that have been documented are related to incorrect lifestyle and nutritional habits, including exercising and walking beyond one's comfort level, vitiated metabolism, dryness in the body and inappropriate meal combination. This includes eating unhealthy meals on a regular basis, eating too much or too little food, eating thick foods, some types of meat, un-boiled milk and curd and eating foods that aggravate *kapha dosha*. Environmental factors, including dust, smoke, wind and cold weather have also been mentioned.

3. Ayurveda conveys that we cannot overlook the underlying cause of the disease being experienced. *Charaka Samhita* states that every illness has a mental cause. Each illness stems from *prajnaparadha* or intellectual failure. Emotional disorders result from forgetting our own genuine soul, tranquillity and peace of mind. *Prajnaparadha* is also brought about by the unproductive and harmful combination of the senses with their respective objects (*asatmyendriyartha*). Asthma is broadly viewed in Ayurveda as a condition that affects several body systems and is marked by a blockage of *prana*, or life force, which makes it difficult or even impossible to breathe. According to the Ayurvedic set of guidelines, this disease poses a grave risk to life. The body's processes cannot operate without *prana*, which can be fatal and create intense fear and worry. The primary contributing factors are regular intake of a poor diet, which weakens digestion and causes the body to produce *ama* (toxic matter).
4. An increase and aggravation in cough (*kasa*) is the sign of *tamaka shvasa*. The primary causes include frequent use of cold water, living in cold and damp environments and coming into touch with air that contains dust, irritating gases, pollens or smoking. Symptoms show up as an increase in undigested materials or toxins (*ama*), diarrhoea, vomiting (*vaman*), poisoning (*visha*), anaemia (*pandu*) and fever (*jwara*) that may be brought on by these circumstances.
5. Based on *doshas*, Ayurveda distinguishes between three forms of asthma:

    - *Vata dosha*, or imbalanced air element, results in the dry kind of asthma.
    - Asthma with aggravated *pitta dosha*, or the fire element, commonly shows up as an infection.
    - As and when there is vitiation and aggravation of *kapha dosha* or the phlegm body humour, asthma is generally of the clogging sort.

- While providing Ayurvedic treatment for asthma, the primary goal is to eradicate the *kapha* in order to alleviate the *shwasavarodha* or restriction of the respiratory path. The *srotosuddhi* method is highlighted for its ability to clear bronchial blockages brought on by *vata dosha* imbalances. Additionally, the *kapha* should be initially liquefied by rubbing the chest with therapeutic oils and *saindhava* (rock salt). It is also advisable to follow a diet and use medications that have the ability to induce mucolysis, or use the *kapha vriddikara dravya*, which facilitates the easy removal of *kapha dosha* obstruction.

Key Takeaways:

- In Ayurveda, when *vayu* (air) moves upwards and constricts the neck and head, it aggravates *kapha* (phlegm), leading to wheezing, dry cough, and spasms. Relief occurs once the phlegm is expelled, temporarily easing the discomfort.
- In Ayurveda, bronchial asthma (*tamaka shwasa*) is described in the *Charaka Samhita*, which categorizes asthma into five types. Among them, *tamaka shwasa*

is difficult to cure but can be controlled, while *ksudra shwasa* is treatable. Poly-herbal combinations are recognized as effective and safe treatments for asthma.

- According to the *Charaka Samhita*, asthma and hiccups are considered highly fatal illnesses, originating from the stomach where *pitta* resides. They result from the simultaneous aggravation of *kapha* and *vata doshas* and negatively affect all tissue components, including the heart.
- In Ayurveda, *vata* and *kapha doshas* contribute to asthma (*shwasa roga*) when *vata* obstructs the channels and circulates through the body. When *kapha* accumulates in the lungs, it thickens and obstructs the bronchial tubes, leading to asthma attacks or difficulty breathing. *vata*'s retrograde movement exacerbates this condition by affecting the neck and head, stimulating *kapha* and causing further blockage and discomfort.
- Asthma treatment in Ayurveda focuses on addressing doshic imbalances and requires the patient to make lifestyle changes, identify emotional triggers, and improve overall immunity. While *panchakarma* (a detoxification process) is the primary treatment, palliative care may be needed for patients who lack the strength for this intensive cleansing. The goal is to remove toxins, enhance disease resistance, and promote a peaceful, balanced life for long-term health.
- The *Charaka Samhita* outlines various causes of health issues that align with modern perspectives, focusing primarily on lifestyle and nutritional habits. Factors like overexercising, poor food choices (e.g., unbalanced meals, thick foods and certain meats),

improper digestion and environmental triggers (such as dust, smoke, wind, and cold weather) are believed to contribute to illness. Additionally, an imbalance in the body's *kapha dosha* is linked to many of these factors.

- Ayurvedic asthma treatment focuses on clearing *kapha* to alleviate respiratory blockages, using methods like *srotosuddhi* and therapies that promote mucolysis and ease *kapha* removal.
-

Chapter 3

OBESITY

Ayurvedic Name: ***Atisthoola, Medho vridhi, Sthaulya***

DISEASE INTRODUCTION

Obesity is a physical condition in which a person experiences an excess of body fat. When an individual is unable to work normally and efficiently and also becomes rather breathless even while talking, this physical condition is termed as obesity.

According to *Bhavaprakasha*, obesity or *medo-roga* sufferer experiences a variety of illnesses. These are:

a. *Kustha* (disease of the skin)
b. *Visarpa* (gangrene or necrosis)
c. *Bhagandara* (ano-fistula)
d. *Jvara* (fever)
e. *Atisara* (diarrhoea)
f. *Prameha* (diabetes)
g. Haemorrhoids (*Arsha*)
h. *Shleepada* (filariasis)
i. *Apachi* (lipomas)
j. *Kamala* (jaundice)
k. *Sweda daurgandha* (a pungent sweat odour)

Ayurvedic Understanding of the Disease

In an obese person, body fat increases and accumulates, *vayu dosha*, or the air that moves inside the obese person's *kosthta* (alimentary canal) moreover augments his/her gastric fire or *jathar agni.* This causes frequent early digestion of food. The obese person often feels more hungry and is also tormented with diverse ailments.

Ayurveda believes that the actual cause of obesity is the impairment of the gastric fire or *agni,* which is responsible for breaking down fat molecules.

However, the main reason for extra fat accumulation in an obese person specified in Ayurveda is lack of exercise and physical exertion, sleeping during the day and consuming more foods in that contain *kapha dosha* or phlegm-increasing properties. As there is an enhancement of sweet juice (*madhur ann-rasa*), it causes an intensification of the *medho-dhatu* (fat body tissue), causing impaired development of other body tissues. As only the fat tissue keeps on increasing in an obese person's body, subsequently, the person suffers from low physical energy,

In the *Ashta Ninditiya* chapter of the *Charaka Samhita*, obesity is described as a condition that can impact a person's overall vitality. The text says that while an obese individual may have a larger body frame, they may experience lower energy levels and a reduced physical endurance. The text also notes that excess weight may lead to a flabby abdomen and chest.

Ayurvedic scriptures like *Charaka Samhita, Sushruta Samhita,* and *Astanga Hridaya* have referred to the disease of obesity as *medoroga* or *sthaulya*. Acharya Charaka recognized eight different types of impediments, or the *ashta nindita purusha.* Of them, *ati sthaulya* (obese individual) is one. The chances of other diseases and disorders like diabetes, cerebro-vascular disease (stroke), hypertension, etc. rise due to obesity and become challenging both to avoid and also cure. Yet, the science of Ayurveda holds immense promise for the prevention and treatment of lifestyle problems such as obesity. According to Ayurveda, obesity or *sthaulya*, is a condition in which the body's *doshas* are aggravated, leading to an inappropriate alteration of nutrition, the development of superfluous *medo-dhatu*, and the incorrect use of nourishment to nurture all other *dhatus* of the body. Therefore, adopting a balanced lifestyle, regular physical activity and controlling stress are essential components of a successful approach to treating and preventing obesity.

Signs and Symptoms

- Excessive body fat and increased body weight, which may, in the long run, impact vital organs, viz. the liver, heart, lungs and kidneys.
- Reduced alertness, both in physical and mental levels, and general impediment.
- Fatty and bulky body stature.
- Lethargy, inactivity and obsessive nature.
- Increased skin fold thickness over the triceps.
- Excessive hunger and thirst.
- Profuse smelling and bodily insufficiency in performing physical activities.

Diet and Lifestyle Management Tips

- Diet control and adequate exercise regime must be followed.
- Conscious restrictions of fatty and sugary foods must be practised, both in amounts and in frequency.
- 3–5 litres of water intake (preferably warm), lemon juice and green leafy vegetables should be increased in diet.
- Fat-enriched and high-calorie food options must be consciously avoided.
- Diet options that include *yavagu* or rice gruel, barley, a bit of honey and fasting is good.
- Rough and easily digestible food items are recommended.
- Slimy foods must be restricted and, at the same time, it is advisable to consume rough foods and grains.
- Overcome laziness and lethargy, avoid sleeping during the day, as well as a sedentary lifestyle.
- Increased indulgence both in physical as well as mental activities and conduct is required.
- Follow regular exercise regimens that induce sweating, along with and Ayurvedic *panchakarma* with extensive options of *vaman, virechana,* and *rakta mokshana* (vomiting, purgative therapies and bloodletting).

Recommended Home Remedies

- Soak 1 tablespoon of *trifla* (the 3 *myrobalans – harad, baheda* and *amla*) powder overnight in water. Take this on empty stomach in the morning.
- Mix half a teaspoon of honey into a glass of warm water, along with a few drops of lemon. Take this in the morning.

Over the world, obesity or *sthaulya*, is becoming more common among people of all ages. *sthaulya* is a *santarpanjanya vyadhi*, according to the Ayurvedic *samhitas*, and it is thoroughly explained in the *Astonindatiya Adhyaya* in *Sutrasthana* of *Charaka Samhita.* In *sthaulya,* mainly the *medovaha srotas* are impacted due to which there is overgrowth of *medo-dhatu*, a process of weight gain that results in obesity. The most affected *srota* in the *sthaulya* disease is *medovaha srota,* which leads to an overgrowth of *medo-dhatu* or the fat tissue.

Vamana and *virechana* are the *Panchakarma* therapies that may be used to treat an *atisthula* (obese person) who is tough and has good stamina. In this case, non-unctuous, warm and potent enemas are advised.

Beverages like honey water and alcoholic concoctions could help reduce extra fat and muscle tissue while balancing the vitiated and aggravated *kapha dosha.*

- Take pure *guggul* (Balsamodendron mukul) in a dose of approx. 15 grains, twice or thrice, along with hot water.
- Groundnut flour is believed to be beneficial for those suffering from obesity. You could mix groundnut flour with wheat flour and make into chapattis.
- Take *shilajit* in the dose of 1–2 grams per day. There are also some formulas, wherein herbs may be added to the same.
- Pure *shilajit* added to *guggul* also proves useful.
- Foods that help decrease *vata* and *kapha doshas* are recommended.
- *Harad* (Terminalia chebula) powder may be used for dry massage on the body.

Ayurvedic management: Line of Treatment with *Shamana* (Palliative) Therapy

- *Ama pachan* (using digestives orally to increase fat metabolism).
- *Ruksha udwartan* (medicated powder massage or *udvartana* because of its qualities, such as *twak prasadakara* (cleanses the skin), *kapha meda vilayana* (liquefies *kapha* and *meda*), *vatahara* (alleviates *vata dosha*) and *angasthirikarana* (provides rigidity to the body).
- Foods and beverages that lower *kapha*, ease *vata* and lessen the *meda dhatu* (fat).
- Following a heavy, yet less nourishing diet and/or foods like salad and honey.
- In addition to physical activity, mental stimulation is advised.

Other Herbs that Help

- *Brahmi* (Centella asiatica)
- Coconut (Cocos nucifera) flowers
- Fresh mango leaves
- Paste of *palash* flowers (Butea monosperma)
- *Tulsi* leaves (holy basil)

Nidana – Causes of Obesity as Discussed in Ayurveda

The following factors contribute to excessive obesity:

- Over-nourishment due to eating heavy, sweet, cold and fatty diet frequently;
- Irregular eating habits;
- Lack of physical activity;

- Abstinence from sexual activity;
- Daytime sleep;
- Uninterrupted happiness;
- Lack of mental activities; and
- Hereditary/genetic imperfection.

These factors could result in a surplus of fat (with extra fat storage) and consequent depletion of other *dhatus*.

Classical Ayurvedic Drugs

- *Arogya vardhani vatti*
- *Yograj guggal*
- *Pushpat rasa*
- *Punarnavaadi mandoor*
- *Pranavallabh rasa*
- *Kchhartamra rasa*
- *Mandoor vatti*
- *Lavangaadi guggulu*
- *Medhohar vidangaadi lauh*
- *Medohar arq*
- *Vyoshaadi guggul*
- *Karpooradya arka*
- *Loha bhasm*
- *Banga bhasm*
- *Vajra bhasm*
- *Khadirarishta*
- *Trifla guggul*
- *Panchtikta ghrit guggul*
- *Amritaadi guggul*
- *Shatavari mandoor*

Panchakarma

Ayurvedic *panchakarma* remedies for obesity include *vaman, virechana,* dry *udvartan*, and *vasti.* In order to promote fat metabolism and lower body weight, dry *udvartan* includes massaging of the body with dry powders. Moreover, weight loss is aided by the removal of excess *kapha* through *vaman* (therapeutic emesis). The purgation therapy, or *virechana*, balances the *pitta dosha* and improves digestion by detoxifying the body. *Vasti* (medicated enemas) aid in the metabolism of fat and balances the *vata dosha.* The goal of these therapies, in addition to following optimum dietary and lifestyle modifications, is to promote general health and maintain sustainable weight loss.

> Acharya Charaka states that the *avarana* (covering) of *vata dosha*, which leads to its aggravation, is caused by fatty tissue obstructing the bodily pathways. The vitiated *vata dosha* primarily travels to the stomach, where it raises the *jathar-agni* (gastric fire). An increase in hunger and quick digestion of food, along with its speedy absorption, is the outcome of the increased digestive fire. Similarly, the subsequent hunger pangs are speedy, making the person want more food. Overindulgence in food leads to an increase in *ahara rasa* production, which, in turn, creates an overabundance of the fat tissue and *sthaulya* or obesity.

Some Ayurvedic facts about Obesity:

1. According to Ayurveda, obesity is defined as an excessive build-up of *mansa* (muscle or flesh) and *meda* (fat/adipose tissue), which causes the hips, abdomen and chest to become flabby. Disorders related to the

metabolism of fat, known as medovushti, may be one of the risk factors for ischemic heart disease (IHD).

- Ancient Ayurveda text describes obesity, or *sthaulya*, as a multidimensional health condition with implications for physical, emotional and psychological well-being. Ayurveda's holistic approach can be used in conjunction with conventional treatments for management of obesity. Effectively addressing and avoiding obesity involves adopting a balanced lifestyle, maintaining physical activity and learning how to manage emotional stress. Seeking individualized counsel and assistance from healthcare professionals and Ayurvedic practitioners is imperative when it comes to managing *sthaulya* safely and efficiently.

2. Due to excessive accumulation of *meda-dhatu* in the body, *vata dosha* acquires blockage to its natural movement and, as a result, *vata* is particularly restricted to the kostha leading to the stimulation of digestive power and absorption of the meal. Because of increased *agni*, a person's digestion increases dramatically, followed by ingestion of larger quantities of food. This person suffers from several severe disorders if they miss meals since it breaks down the *dhatus*. The two most problematic and complex elements are *agni* and *vata*, which burn an obese person like a forest fire. When there is an extreme build-up of fat, aggravated and imbalanced *vata* and *agni* can cause serious illnesses. In extreme cases, it may prove fatal, too.

3. Obesity has existed for as long as humanity, according to ancient Ayurvedic texts. Because of the similar features between them, Acharya Charaka states that the continuous use of the causative components aggravates *meda dhatu* and *kapha dosha*, causing the aggravated *meda* to obstruct the *srotas* (functional channels) and lead to obesity. He also mentions that the most hazardous ailment is *sthaulya*.

   The eight characteristics of overweight individuals are as follows:

   - Lower life expectancy;
   - Disordered mobility;
   - Difficulty engaging in sexual activity;
   - General debility;
   - Body odour originating;
   - Heavy sweating;
   - Excessive consumption of food or drink; and
   - Hypertension.

4. According to Ayurveda, obesity or *sthaulya* is caused by an imbalance in the body's *doshas*, especially the *vata* and *kapha*. Managing obesity is trickier due to this *dosha* combination. Sedentary lifestyle, poor eating patterns and psychological variables are some of the causes that lead to the build-up of extra fat. Ayurveda focusses on the body's flexibility of the fatty tissue rather than just weight in kilograms. An unhealthy diet causes the body to accumulate adipose tissue, which causes weight gain and obesity. Exercise reduces the energy imbalance that leads to weight growth and obesity by

balancing the amount of calories spent and absorbed. In Ayurveda, treating obesity involves more than just losing weight; it also takes into account modifying the metabolic processes by getting rid of excess fat and *ama*, which helps balance the role of *kapha* and avoid aggravating the *vata*. Sturdy tissues and an enhanced digestive fire are considered essential as these indicate proper metabolism. In addition, Ayurveda prescribes yoga and food plans to help with weight loss and the management of obesity.

5. In Ayurveda, the five-step *panchakarma* therapy is incredibly effective at eliminating toxins from the body while treating obesity-related illnesses. Several *panchakarma* therapies, such as *virechana* or purgation therapy, *basti* or medicated enema and deep tissue massages, such as *mardanam* and *udwarthanam*, are recommended, particularly for weight loss treatment in Ayurveda. Herbal powders and oils are used in *mardanam* and *udwarthanam* massages to relieve stiffness in the body and clear any obstructions. Also, while giving a massage, sesame seed oil (*til taila*) can be used with other herbs to encourage supple skin and minimize adipose tissues. These oil massages cause the body's pores to open up, raising tissue temperature and promoting fat metabolism in the obese person making *panchakarma* Ayurvedic weight-loss treatment more accepted and authentic.
6. The serious disease known as obesity is caused by dietary imbalance that result in abnormal adipose tissue growth and increase in body weight. According to Acharya Charaka, obesity falls under the category of

ashtaninditiya purusha in Ayurveda. Both Ayurveda and yoga largely emphasize the spiritual and mental aspects of healing. In addition to optimum *ahara* (planned diet) and *vihara* (lifestyle adjustment) for the management of obesity, *udwarthana*, *shodhana* and *shamana chikitsa* are recommended.

- The objective of Ayurveda is to avoid disease and, by and large, promote the well-being of an individual. It heals illnesses based on the *doshas* and *dushya*, which are crucial factors in the onset of any illness. In case of sthulya, the *kapha vata doshas* and *rasa*, *mamsa* and *medha dhatus* are the primary vitiated *doshas* and dushyas, respectively. Ayurveda outlines the most fundamental course of treatment as *nidana parivarjana*, or avoiding the cause i.e. sedentary lifestyle, sleeping during the day and not exercising, which causes an abnormal build-up of *medha dhatu*, or fat, in the body.

Key Takeaways:

- In Ayurveda, obesity is caused by an imbalance in the gastric fire (*agni*), which fails to break down fat properly, leading to increased hunger and accumulation of body fat. The *vayu dosha*'s disturbance further aggravates digestion, resulting in frequent hunger and various health issues.
- Ayurveda describes obesity (*medoroga* or *sthaulya*) as a condition resulting from imbalanced *doshas*, improper nutrition, and excessive fat accumulation. It can lead

to serious diseases like diabetes and hypertension, but Ayurveda offers effective prevention and treatment through a balanced lifestyle, regular exercise, and stress management.

- Obesity (*sthaulya*) is a condition caused by an imbalance in the *medovaha srotas*, leading to excess fat tissue (*medo-dhatu*). Ayurvedic treatments, such as *vamana* and *virechana*, along with specific beverages like honey water and alcohol concoctions, can help reduce excess fat and balance *kapha dosha*.
- Ayurvedic *panchakarma* therapies for obesity, including *vaman*, *virechana*, dry *udvartan*, and *vasti*, aim to detoxify the body, balance *doshas*, and promote fat metabolism. These treatments, combined with dietary and lifestyle changes, support sustainable weight loss and overall health.
- Ayurveda views obesity (*sthaulya*) as a complex condition affecting physical, emotional, and psychological well-being. A holistic approach that includes a balanced lifestyle, physical activity, and stress management, along with professional guidance, is essential for effective and safe obesity management.
- Ancient Ayurvedic texts recognize obesity as a long-standing condition, attributing it to the aggravation of *meda dhatu* and *kapha dosha*, which obstruct the *srotas* (functional channels), leading to obesity. Acharya Charaka highlights *sthaulya* as one of the most hazardous ailments.
- *Panchakarma* therapy is highly effective for treating obesity-related illnesses by eliminating toxins and promoting weight loss. Techniques like *virechana*

(purgation), *basti* (medicated enema), and deep tissue massages (*mardanam, udwarthanam*) using herbal oils help clear obstructions, improve metabolism, and reduce adipose tissue.

Chapter 4

HEART DISEASE

Ayurvedic Name: ***Hridroga***

All ailments that particularly arise in the heart are referred to as heart disease, wherein changes are found in the heartbeat or the sound becoming either dull or intense. There is decreased or no supply of oxygen and nutrient-rich blood to the heart muscle by the coronary artery which results in the production of diseases like angina, myocardial infarction and coronary artery disease.

Ayurvedic Understanding of the Disease

Heart disease is termed as *hridroga* in Ayurveda text. It manifests itself due to imbalance and vitiation in the *vata dosha*, although heart disease may result from imbalance in either or all of the three *doshas vata, pitta*, and *kapha*.

Vitiation in the air body humour causes a disruption in the *rasa dhatu* of the body, which further causes heart disease. Any vitiation in the three body humours, viz. air, fire and phlegm, or a collective distortion of all the humours is believed to be the basis of heart disease.

Signs and Symptoms

Decreased or no supply of oxygen and nutrient-rich blood to the heart muscle by the coronary artery results in diseases like angina, myocardial infarction and coronary artery disease. Perhaps, there is congenital or acquired disease/s of the endocardium, myocardium and pericardium.

Ayurveda concept of disease evaluation pertains to an imbalanced approach to diet and lifestyle. The consumption of an incompatible diet is considered highly imperative in the formation of heart disease. Improper everyday lifestyle fortified with increasing stress and strain add to the ailment. Ayurveda strongly emphasizes the merits of consciously acknowledging *ahara* (balanced diet) and *vihara* (the right lifestyle). These are the two main factors that may help you avoid heart disease.

Vata Dosha Imbalance of the Heart

This is termed as *vataja* or *vatik hridya roga* in Ayurveda. In this particular ailment, there is dilatation of the heart along with painful sensations like breaking, cutting with an axe or piercing of a needle etc. *Vata* symptoms of heart disease generally emerge as palpitations and arrhythmia.

Pitta Dosha Imbalance of the Heart

This is referred to as *pittaja* or *paittik hridya roga* in Ayurveda. Along with augmented heat sensation, there is fainting, increased sweating, dryness of the mouth and a feeling of fumes

In Ayurveda, cardiovascular disorders are addressed and explored in relation to *Hridroga*. Numerous herbs and herbal supplements support the management and prevention of cardiovascular disease. In the context of *Hridroga*, Ayurveda offers an alternative interpretation of the etio-pathogenesis of such illnesses and the subsequent treatment. Ancient Ayurvedic remedies for heart disease provide relevant validity for the treatment and prevention of cardiovascular diseases. Ayurvedic medications, herbs and medicinal plants all have anti-hyper-lipidemic, anti-platelet aggregation, blood pressure-lowering, anti-atherogenic and effective cardio-protective qualities. To avoid heart disease, it is advised that we maintain a balanced diet, engage in optimal and regular exercise, abstain from alcohol and tobacco use and learn stress management techniques. When used to treat conditions like cardiovascular disease (CVD), scientific knowledge of numerous clinical factors can have a profound positive impact on both the preventive and curative elements of cardiovascular diseases.

emerging from the mouth cavity. While the pain in the heart region may feel like forceful sucking, the individual experiences burning sensitivity and unquenched thirst. Generally the *pitta* symptoms of heart disease emerge as angina. Also, there could be yellow colouration when the liver is congested by heart failure.

Kapha Dosha Imbalance on the Heart

Expressed in Ayurveda as *kaphaja* or *shleshmik hridya roga,* there is heaviness in the heart region, along with loss of hunger, diminished gastric fire and occasional indigestion, as well as phlegm in the mouth with sweet taste. *Kapha* symptoms of heart disease generally emerge as drowsiness and a heavy sensation in the heart.

***Tri-Doshas* (*Vata, Pitta* and *Kapha*) Imbalance of the Heart**

Tridoshaja hridroga shows combined symptoms of an imbalance in all the three *doshas*, viz. *vata, pitta* and *kapha doshas.* It has also been mentioned that taking more of jaggery or *gur*, milk and milk products or *til* (sesame seeds) may result in the formation of a cyst or abscess (swelling) in the heart region. Moreover, the flow of mucous tissue and *rasa* (juice) is enhanced, which produces of *krimi* (worms) in the heart causing a severely painful condition, like the piercing of a needle, in the heart region.

Worm Infestation in the Heart

Termed as *krimija hridroga* in Ayurveda, there is a precise amalgamation of signs like yawning, feeling of nausea and vomiting, intense mucous production in the mouth, piercing painful sensation, dizziness, loss of hunger, darkened eyes, as well as darkness before the eyes and emaciation.

Diet and Lifestyle Management Tips

- In diet, consuming simple, wholesome, easily digestible and fat-free foods is recommended.
- Fruit and vegetable juices are good.
- Salt intake must be less; refrain from eating highly spicy, fried foods and excessively sugars diet items.
- Less physical exertion is advisable; however, leisurely walks in fresh air and sunbathing are equally helpful.
- Keeping a relaxed mental outlook and reducing mental stress and strain are necessary.

Ayurveda believes that all actions within the body, whether voluntary or involuntary, are governed by the *vata dosha.* Also, it is obvious that the actions involved in the natural physiological calls or bodily urges, are involuntary, but these are partially under voluntary control.

Classical texts from Ayurveda state that such natural urges should be strictly attended to without disturbing their natural flow. Some urges can be intentionally or inadvertently initiated (*udirana*) or suppressed (*dhaaran*), redirecting the normal flow of *vayu*, thus leaving scope for severe morbidities in the heart, eventually causing cardiovascular disorders (CVD). Although, since *vata dosha* has unique attributes of *vega* (locomotion) that moves in a specific direction, its intensities can be quantified with the help of modern techniques.

Recommended Home Remedies

- Swallow 2–4 cloves of garlic, on empty stomach, in the morning.
- Take clove powder two times a day.
- Make a powder of *ajwain* and *hing* – to be taken twice after meals with water.
- Pound some bark of Arjun and take the powder in a dose of half to 1 teaspoon, twice, along with milk or water.
- Take 1 teaspoonful of the powder of Arjun bark. Boil it in a mixture of 1 cup milk and 1 cup water till half remains. Take this twice a day.
- Make a cinnamon powder and take it twice a day. This acts as a heart tonic and also helps to lower elevated cholesterol levels.
- Take 1 cup juice of freshly ground gourd. To this, add 7–8 leaves each of *tulsi* and mint. Take the mixture twice.

- Massage the chest with eucalyptus oil.
- Asparagus is believed to be virtuous for the heart. A regular intake in the form of powder (3–5 grams) or juice (10–20 ml) is recommended for heart patients. This is because it is believed to improve the overall functioning of the vital organ.
- You can prepare another easy remedy at home. Pound equal quantities of dried *amla* and *mishri* together. Take 1–2 teaspoons of the mixture twice a day, along with water, for strengthening the heart.
- Grapes are also recommended for those suffering from heart disease. This is because being soft, slimy and cold by nature, grapes have a soothing and calming effect on the nervous system.
- A decoction prepared by boiling approx. 1–2 teaspoons of dried ginger is to be taken warm, once or twice in a day's time.
- Betel is also believed to be good for the heart and is used to cure heart ailments. Fresh juice extracted by pounding betel leaves can be taken twice in a dose of approx. 1–2 teaspoons.
- A *murabba* (sweet jelly) of apple and carrot is recommended as a heart tonic.
- A moderate intake of ripe mango strengthens the heart and provides relief from palpitations.

Other Herbs that Help

- Cardamom (Elettaria cardamomum)
- Black pepper
- *Kushmanda* (Benincasa hispida)
- Clove (Syzygium aromaticum)

- *Sarapgandha* (Rawolfia serpentina)
- *Brahmi* (Centella asiatica)
- *Shatavari* (Asparagus racemosus)
- Coconut (Cocos nucifera) flowers
- Fresh mango leaves
- Paste of *palash* flowers (Butea monosperma)
- *Tulsi* Leaves (holy basil)
- Groundnut flour
- *Dalchini* (Cinnamomum zeylanicum)
- *Arjuna* (Terminalia arjuna)

While hereditary factors can contribute to heart diseases, poor nutrition and lifestyle options are the major sources of heart disease aggravation. The goal of Ayurvedic remedies for heart disease is to pinpoint the underlying cause of the condition and provide a customized remedy. Although genetics plays some role in heart diseases, the majority of heart diseases become aggravated because of wrong lifestyle choices and incorrect diet. Ayurveda treatment emphasize the identification of the basic grounds of the heart disease and offers a personalized resolution for the problem.

Ayurveda helps assist and balance the vitiated *doshas* and avoid heart disease. The three *doshas* – *vata, pitta* and *kapha* – when aggravated and vitiated, can lay the foundation of a heart disease.

- Aggravated *vata dosha* can raise heart rate and blood pressure in addition to disrupting the cardiac rhythm.
- Elevated *pitta* can lead to a burning sensation and weaken the heart's resistance to emotional hazards.
- Elevated *kapha* in the body can aggravate cholesterol and cause heart blockages.

Classical Ayurvedic Drugs

- *Abhrak bhasm*
- *Hridyarnava rasa*
- *Swarna bhasm*
- *Lakshmi narayan rasa*
- *Shila sindur rasa*
- *Arjunarishta*
- *Ahifenasava*
- *Hridyarnava rasa*
- *Swarna Vasant malti rasa*
- *Arjun quath*
- *Arjun ghrit*
- *Mukta bhasm*
- *Karpooradya arka*
- *Hridyavirechana leha*
- *Saptavimashtika guggul*
- *Shring bhasm*
- *Brihat saindhavaadi taila*
- *Saptasara kwath churan*
- *Sarpgandhaghan vatti*
- *Praval pishti*
- *Mukta pishti*

PANCHAKARMA

Panchakarma therapy for heart disease is carefully considered in Ayurveda. Due to its strength, *vaman* (therapeutic emesis) should usually be avoided or taken up only under the guidance of a professional. On the other hand, purgation therapy, or *virechana*, is recommended to reduce inflammation and balance *pitta dosha* while detoxifying the body. It is also advised to use *vasti* (medicated enemas) to balance the *vata dosha* and enhance general cardiovascular health. Together with sensible dietary and lifestyle changes, these therapies can promote heart health when used judiciously.

> *Rasa dhatu dushti* or vitiated *rasa dhatu* is one among many clinical constructs mentioned in Ayurveda that need to be inferred through observable clinical features. Ayurveda believes that, in heart diseases, there is a prevalence of *rasa dhatu dushti* more than all other *dhatus* or tissues (functionally distinct body elements). From the Ayurvedic perspective, it can be observed that CVD as well as present-day lifestyle disorders are *santarpanothavyadhis* (diseases caused by over-nutrition). Excessive energy intake (*atipurana*), along with a sedentary lifestyle (*avyayama*) lead to deranged metabolism of the macronutrients, mainly carbohydrates and fats. Such factors have been considered, in Ayurveda, as definite causes leading to *rasa dhatu dushti* and the heart disease.

Some Ayurvedic facts on Heart Disease:

1. In Ayurveda, cardiovascular disorders are regarded as *hridroga*. Numerous herbs and herbal supplements support the management and prevention of cardiovascular disease. In the context of *hridroga*, Ayurveda offers an alternative interpretation of the etio-pathogenesis of heart ailments. Herbs and nutritional supplements can play a big part in cardiac disease prevention. A number of Ayurvedic medications, herbs and medicinal plants have anti-hyperlipidemic, anti-platelet aggregation, blood pressure-lowering, anti-atherogenic and valuable cardio-protective qualities.

To avoid heart disease, it is advised that we also maintain a balanced diet, engage in optimal and regular exercise and abstain from alcohol and tobacco use. Moreover, we must gain essential knowledge of stress management techniques. When used to treat conditions like cardiovascular disease (CVD), scientific knowledge from the ancient Ayurveda text, citing numerous clinical factors, can have a profound positive impact on both the preventive and curative elements of heart diseases.

2. There are five different types of heart disease as identified in the authentic writings according to the *doshas* in Ayurveda, which are *vataja*, *pittaja*, *kaphaja*, *sannipathaja* and *krimija*. These diseases are characterized by pain, burning sensation, phlegm production, combinations of all the three and bacterial infections, respectively.

    - *Doshas* (*vata, pitta* and *kapha*) are vitiated due to overeating excessive consumption of hot and heavy foods, as well as astringent and bitter foods. Consuming food before the previous meal is digested is another factor, wherein a large amount of physical strain is experienced, emotional feelings are suppressed, and natural urges are not followed.
    - *Vataja Hridroga's* etiological components are clearly stated and elucidated in Ayurveda as this heart disease is believed to be primarily caused due to the vitiation of the *vata dosha*, which involves heart functions. Sorrow (*shoka*), fasting (*upavasa*), excessive exercise (*vyayama*) and unwholesome eating (*alp-bojanni*) all contribute to this disease.

3. Ayurveda acknowledges that *vyana-vayu* governs both the movement of the heart and valvular abnormalities. Presumably, *meda dhatu* (fat tissue) gives rise to the pericardium, *manasa dhatu* (muscle tissue) to the myocardium and *rasa* and *rakta* (juice and blood) to the endocardium. Maintaining vitiated *rasa* and *rakta* circulating in the endocardium might lead to a progressive development of valvular inflammation, which eventually progresses to further infectious condition and eventually results in the formation of *krimis* (worms or bacterial infection). When *mansadusti* (discrepancy of the muscle tissue) persists in this condition for an extended length of time, valves deteriorate and valvular diseases, such as regurgitation and stenosis, arise. A murmur is a defining characteristic of valvular heart disease. This is considered primarily a rheumatic disease. In Ayurveda, this could be regarded as *amavata*'s synonym. Therefore, the primary goal of the treatment for relieving heart disease is to address the imbalanced *vata*, *rasa*, *rakta* and *mamsa*.
4. One of the basic patho-physiological entities in the human body, *vata dosha* has distinct and ever-changing qualities. *Vayu* or the *vata dosha* governs all internal bodily movements, both voluntary and involuntary. Also, a number of natural physiological calls and impulses cause actions that are partially under human control but mainly involuntary. Such natural urges should be properly adhered to without interfering with their natural flow, according to traditional Ayurvedic teachings. Although, certain desires can be deliberately or unintentionally moved or subdued, which can re-

route the natural *vayu* flow and create serious cardiac morbidities that lead to cardiovascular disease (CVD). It is *vata*'s extraordinary ability to move in a single direction (locomotion) and its intensities can be calculated using contemporary methods. And yet, they can be effectively taken care of with Ayurvedic medicines. Many formulations are portrayed in Ayurvedic classics for this purpose. The treatment modality in *vataja hridroga*, as described in Ayurveda, which simulates pain, is similar to ischemic heart diseases.

5. Ayurvedic treatments are endowed with *rasayanas* as brain rejuvenation remedies that strengthen the brain to manage stressful situations effectively, which, in due course, help to prevent heart disease. Also, according to Ayurveda, having strong digestion (*agni*) and no toxins (*ama*) are essential for maintaining heart health. Ayurveda aids in taking care of *agni* and *ama* issues. Eventually, *ojas* is created by the potent *agni*, which is a philosophy that is preserved in the science of Ayurveda. It is strongly believed that an individual with great immunity and endurance is also peaceful and content. This person also has a healthy and robust *ojas*, which is the essence of all *dhatus* or tissues. At the same time, it strengthens the emotion – considered vital in Ayurveda. This is because anger, grief and resentment are examples of pent-up emotions that are bad and futile for the heart. In Ayurveda, all unpleasant emotions are classified as tamasic. *Tamasic* emotions can be banished and rather the *satvic* emotions can be developed with the aid of Ayurvedic herbs for the heart, and practising yoga and pranayama.

6. According to Acharya Sushruta, in the presence of the etiological factors all the three *doshas* get vitiated and provoked, spread out of their areas and vitiate the *rasa dhatu* in the heart. The manifestation of a vitiated *rasa dhatu* (lymph/chyle) lays the ground for various types of pain, which is called *hridbadha* or *hridroga*. Improper diet (excessive intake of *kshar*, salty or *lavana rasa*, *virudahbhojana* or incompatible food intake) and *vegadharna* (holding on to bodily urges), *chinta*, *krodha* (mental emotions of worry and anger) etc. are a few among the many causes of *Hridroga*. In understanding the symptomology of cardiovascular disorder, *vaivarnya* (*panduta/shweta/shyava*) can be correlated to pallor and cyanosis, *murcchato* to syncope, *kasato* to cough with or without hemoptysis, *shwasato* or breathlessness or dyspnoea, *ruja* to chest pain or discomfort. Drugs used in various formulations in *Hridroga* have properties like *pachana*, *deepana*, *hridya*, *anulomana*, *rasayana* and *krimihara*.

KEY TAKEAWAYS:

- Heart disease, or *hridyroga*, in Ayurveda is caused by an imbalance in the *vata dosha*, although it can result from disturbances in *vata*, *pitta* and *kapha doshas*. Vitiation in these *doshas*, especially in the air (*vata*), disrupts the *rasa dhatu* and leads to heart disease.
- Ayurveda offers a unique approach to cardiovascular disorders (*hridroga*), focusing on herbs and remedies with anti-hyperlipidemic, anti-platelet, blood pressure-lowering and cardio-protective properties. Prevention

and treatment emphasize a balanced diet, regular exercise, stress management, and avoiding alcohol and tobacco use for optimal heart health.

- *Tridoshaja hridroga* in Ayurveda involves an imbalance of *vata, pitta,* and *kapha doshas,* leading to symptoms like swelling or cyst formation in the heart. Overconsumption of jaggery, milk, and sesame seeds can contribute to this, along with enhanced mucous flow, causing severe pain due to the formation of *krimi* (worms) in the heart.
- Ayurveda asserts that *vata dosha* governs both voluntary and involuntary bodily actions, including natural urges. Disrupting or suppressing these urges can disturb the flow of *vayu*, leading to serious health issues like cardiovascular disorders. Modern techniques can help quantify the intensity of *vata*'s influence on the body.
- Ayurveda emphasizes that heart disease is primarily driven by poor lifestyle and diet, despite some genetic influence. Treatment focuses on balancing the vitiated *doshas* – *vata*, *pitta*, and *kapha* – to address the root cause of the condition. *Vata* can disrupt heart rate, *pitta* affects emotional resilience, and *kapha* contributes to cholesterol buildup and blockages.
- Ayurvedic treatments focus on rejuvenating the brain with *rasayanas* to manage stress and prevent heart disease. A strong *agni* (digestion) and elimination of *ama* (toxins) are crucial for heart health. By promoting *ojas* (vital energy) and fostering satvic emotions, Ayurveda strengthens immunity and emotional balance, which are key for heart vitality.

Chapter 5

CERVICAL SPONDYLOSIS

Ayurvedic Name: ***Griva Sandhigata Vata, Manyastambh***

Disease Introduction:

This disease is a form of arthritis of the cervical vertebrae that affects the neck region and the connecting bony, muscular and ligament structure. There is acute pain and stiffness in the neck area and around the shoulders, radiating to the back. There may also be giddiness and difficulty in neck movement.

Ayurvedic Understanding of the Disease

Vitiation or aggravation in the *vata* and *kapha doshas* or body humours is believed to be the predisposing cause. There is rigidity of the neck muscle along with pain and stiffness in the back of the neck, arms and shoulders.

Vata, the main *dosha* for movement, makes the major portion of the skeleto-muscular system and the nervous system; and therefore, the health issues that relate to these body systems are largely caused by aggravated and imbalanced *vata dosha.* Cervical Spondylosis may be considered one among the *vata vyadhis.*

Cervical spondylosis is a chronic degenerative disease of the cervical spine, referred to in Ayurveda as *greeva stambha,* which is principally a *vata dosha* health issue. This is because, according to Ayurveda, movement of the body is considered to be caused mainly by the *vyana vata.* Generally, for the treatment of *vata-vyadhis,* it has been suggested to take to the therapies of oleation (*snehana*) and steam fomentation (*swedana*). In ancient Ayurveda, it is mentioned that *vakra* and *stabdha* (stiffened) body parts (as the neck is in cervical spondylosis) can be made *namayita* (bent lightly) by combining the processes of *snehana* and *swedana.* Additionally, the effects of these karmas aid the body's tissues (*dhatus*) to be nourished, the *agni-bala* (gastric fire) to be amplified and, eventually, the body to become stronger and healthier.

Signs and Symptoms

- There is pain and stiffness in the neck, shoulder and arms.
- Neck move,ents may be restricted.
- There may also be giddiness or vertigo upon touching the chin to the chest.
- The pain tends to aggravate with spinal movements.
- Memory loss and insomnia may result.

Diet and Lifestyle Management Tips

- Include *katu rasa* (bitter taste) in diet, such as bitter gourd, *neem,* etc.
- Restrict the consumption of sour foods.

- Avoid refined foods and refined flour (*maida*).
- Neck exercises help.
- Using a hard bed without a pillow, or with only a soft pillow, is recommended.
- Avoid forceful neck exercises.
- Hot fomentation of the neck area is recommended for about 15–30 minutes a day. Use a tolerably hot salt poultice in a cotton cloth for this purpose.
- Avoid any form of violent massage techniques and applying pressure in the neck region.
- A warmed sand-poultice may be used for local application.
- Yoga asanas like *Padmasana, Gomukh Asana, Sidhasana* and *Vajrasana* are helpful.
- Gentle massage of the neck and shoulders using warm mustard oil mixed with camphor (*kapur*) also helps.

As per Ayurveda, by applying *vatahara* oils locally and taking oral *vatahara* treatment, inflammation is significantly reduced. This is because by providing steam, muscle spasms are reduced. This, in turn, facilitates improved blood supply and better nerve transmission to the affected region, leading to symptomatic progress.

The *vatahara* therapy, Ayurvedic medicine or herbs for combating *vata*, *vata*-supressing *taila* for topical application and *nadi sweda* (local steam with *vata*-controlling herbal *kwatha* or decoction) are recommended for easing *greeva stambha*. This is due to Ayurveda's belief that vitiated *vata dosha* is the cause of *stambha* and *shoola* (pain and stiffness). Therefore, *vata dosha*-suppressing/balancing oil, or *taila,* used topically, and *guggulu* preparation, taken orally, both aid in correcting *vata* vitiation.

Recommended Home Remedies

- Mix raw turmeric powder (1 teaspoon) and dried ginger powder (1/4 teaspoon) in a glass of warm milk and drink it at bedtime.
- Tenderly massage the back of the neck with previously warmed sesame seed oil or mustard oil. Any medicated muscle relaxant oil or balm also helps.
- Hot fomentation of the neck region with the help of sand or salt poultice is useful.
- Prepare a decoction of dried ginger and add some pure castor oil. Take this warm (approx. half cup) at bedtime.
- Dissolve some camphor in mustard oil and warm the same. Apply on the site of pain.
- Neck exercises and mild acupressure play a good role in curing this disease.
- Massage the back of the neck with dried ginger powder mixed in previously warmed mustard oil for relief. It is advisable to apply hot fomentation afterwards.

Other Herbs that Help:

- *Haldi* (Turmeric)
- *Harsingaar*
- *Lahsun* (Garlic)
- *Gehun ke jware* (Sprouted wheat)
- *Methi-dana* (Soaked fenugreek seeds)

Classical Ayurvedic Drugs:

- *Yograj guggul*
- *Maha yograj guggul*
- *Maha narayan taila*

- *Krishna chaturmukh rasa*
- *Vat gtankush rasa*
- *Sihnad guggul*
- *Kalpatru nasya*
- *Brihat vat chintamani rasa*
- *Rasa sindhur + Sunthi churan*
- *Shudh kuchla + Vat gajankush rasa*
- *Trifla churan*
- *Panchmoola kwatha*
- *Dashmool kwath with pushkarmoola*
- *Brihat saindhavaadi taila (local massage)*
- *Kalpatru nasya*

Panchakarma

Nasya and *vasti* are two Ayurvedic *panchakarma* treatments for cervical spondylosis. Medicated oils are used in *nasya* (nasal administration) to unclog nasal passages, ease tension in the neck and reduce the inflammation. Also, by balancing the *vata dosha, vasti* (medicated enemas) relieves stiffness and pain in the cervical area. The goal of these treatments is to lessen the pain, increase the range of motion, especially in the neck region, and support spinal health in general. Specific workouts and nutrition advice are added to these treatments to maximize their therapeutic effects.

Some Ayurvedic facts about Cervical Spondylosis

1. Cervical Spondylosis is referred to as *manyastambh* in Ayurveda. This term is derived from the words *manya*, meaning nape of the neck, and *stambh*, meaning stiffness or rigidity. In this disease, it is believed that

As per Ayurveda, *vyana vayu* governs the body's movements, and cervical spondylosis is regarded as similar to *greeva stambha*, which is a *vata* condition.

Common symptoms are headaches, neck pain while moving the head, tingling or numbness in the affected arm, with or without paralysis, and even vertigo. Ayurvedic medicine improves this condition by reducing both the inflammation as well as spasms through the use of *nadi sweda* (local heat) and *vatahara* treatment.

These manifestations have been treated with a variety of Ayurvedic therapies that aid in managing cervical spondylosis with the recommended Ayurvedic medications, as well as *Panchakarma* treatments.

vata takes shelter in the *snayu* (ligaments) of the *manyapradesh*, or the neck. It is characterized by properties of *guru* (heaviness), *stambha* (rigidity) in the neck region mentioned as *manyapradesha*, *ruk* (pain) and *chestastambh* (rigidnesss). The clinical presentation of *manyastambh* resembles the disease of cervical spondylosis. It is a type of *vatavyadhi* (disease due to the vitiation of *vata dosha*). It can occur as *nanatmaja vikara* and the treatment procedure described in Ayurveda focusses not only on medicines but also lifestyle alteration, therefore comprising a holistic approach in the management of cervical spondylosis.

2. According to Ayurveda, the issues that are associated with *greeva stambha*, or cervical spondylosis, are: *bhrama* (vertigo) and *bahu-shosha* (upper limb weakness and emaciation). In *nanatamaj vata-vyadhi*, all of these symptoms are taken into account (disorders

that are attributable to *vata dosha*). Whereas *bhrama* is caused by an unbalanced *pitta* and *vata dosha*, *bahushosha* may result from vitiated *vata* and deficient *kapha dosha*.

- *Vata* is vitiated by a number of etiological factors, including *dhatukshaya* (depletion of bodily tissue) and *margavarana* (obstruction in the natural route of *vata* such as in case of normal circulation, combination of tissue elements, etc.). Thus, in a vicious cycle, vitiated *vata* results in *margavarana* and *dhatukshaya*, and may cause the symptoms of cervical spondylosis. Due to vitiated *vata dosha*, *sthanik kapha* (localized *kapha dosha* present in the cervical area) is also depleted.
- The core categories of Ayurvedic *samprapti* (pathology) comprise all forms of cervical spondylosis disease. *Dhatukshaya* is treated with *brihmana* (nutrition). Therefore, in cervical spondylosis, *snigdha* (unctuous), *srotosodhaka* (bio-purification of micro-channels), *vatanulomaka* (correction of *vata dosha* function) treatments and management, which is compatible with *kapha* and *pitta doshas*, should be used.

3. For relieving *greeva stambha*, the *vatahara* treatment viz. Ayurvedic medicines for local intake and application of recommended *vata*-suppressing *taila* for local use along with *nadi sweda* (local steam) are advised. This is because Ayurveda believes that *stambha* and *shoola* (stiffness and pain) are caused by vitiated *vata dosha*.

Thus, these Ayurvedic *vata*-suppressing therapies and application or local massage of *vatahara taila* help to correct the *vata* vitiation. Moreover, *guggul* is the suggested herb of choice, as indicated in *Vatavyadhi Chikitsa* by Acharya Charaka. Besides, *nadi sweda* provides ushan *upachara* (hot fomentation) locally. Furthermore, the *snehana* and *swedana* processes result in the suppression of *vata*. The *snigdha* and *ushna gunas* (oily and hot properties) of *snehana* and *swedana karmas* work remarkably against the *ruksha* and *sheeta gunas* (rough and cold properties) of *vata dosha*.

4. Charaka has mentioned *guggulu* in *Vatavyadhi Chikitsa*. Additionally, *nadisweda* provides local *ushna upachara*, or heat treatment. All kinds of *snehana swedana* lead to *vata* suppression. The *ruksha* and *sheeta gunas* of *vata* are opposed by the *snigdha* and *ushna gunas* of *snehana swedana*.

    - Additionally, inflammation is decreased by administering *vatahara* therapy orally and topically. Administering steam helps to ease muscle spasms. When the inflammation and spasms are reduced, the afflicted area receives better blood flow and nerve conduction, which provides clinical relief and, eventually, functional status in cases of cervical spondylosis. Various Ayurvedic treatments have been recommended for this disease with a combination of *panchakarma* procedures and Ayurvedic oral medications especially for relieving *greeva stambha* (neck stiffness).

5. In case of those suffering from cervical spondylosis,

there is vitiation of *vata dosha*, which further causes *stambha* and *shoola* (pain and stiffness). *vata* vitiation may be corrected by taking Ayurvedic medicines orally, like *guggulu* preparations, and also local application of *vatahara* (*vata* suppressing) *taila* or a warm oil. Additionally, *nadisweda* (local heat) provides local *ushna upachara*, or heat treatment. The most commonly experienced symptoms in individuals with cervical spondylosis are headache, neck pain, tingling or numbness, with or without arm weakness, and dizziness. Since nerve compression and muscular spasms cause this disease's symptoms, *vatahara* reduction of inflammation and spasms is recommended in Ayurveda therapies.

6. In Ayurvedic medicine, the *vatahara* treatment – which involves consuming *guggulu* preparation orally, applying *vatahara taila* topically and administering steam with *vata*-suppressing decoctions – is advised as a means of treating cervical spondylosis, also known as *greeva stambha*. Additionally, by using *vatahara* oils topically and taking *vatahara* treatment internally, inflammation may be reduced significantly, and muscle spasms eased by applying steam. As a result of the decreased inflammation and spasm, the affected area receives better blood flow and nerve transmission, which brings clinical relief and, in the end, the functional status of the person suffering from the disease of cervical spondylosis improves.
7. In Ayurveda, the phrase *manyastambh* refers to cervical spondylosis. *Manya* stands for nape of the neck, while *stambh* implies firmness or rigidity.

- Properties like *stambha* (rigidity) in the neck region, *ruk* (pain), *chestastambh* (inflexibility) and *guru* (heaviness) define this physical condition. The clinical manifestation of cervical spondylosis is similar to that of *manyastambha*. This kind of illness is called *vata-vyadhi*, or vitiation of the *vata dosha*. Both *kaphavruta vata* and *nanatmaja vikara* may occur. The Ayurvedic treatment protocol for this illness emphasizes on lifestyle modification in addition to medication, thus taking a holistic approach to disease management.

Key Takeaways:

- Cervical spondylosis (*greeva stambha*) is linked to *vata dosha* imbalances in Ayurveda. Treatment involves therapies like oleation (*snehana*) and steam fomentation (*swedana*) to soften stiff body parts, nourish tissues, enhance digestive fire (*agni*), and promote overall health and strength.
- In Ayurveda, treating cervical spondylosis (*greeva stambha*) involves *vatahara* therapies like *vata*-suppressing oils and oral herbs (e.g., *guggulu*) to reduce inflammation, ease muscle spasms, and restore blood flow. Local steam treatment (*nadi sweda*) with herbal decoctions supports nerve function and relieves pain and stiffness caused by *vata* imbalances.
- *Nasya* (nasal administration of medicated oils) and *vasti* (medicated enemas) are Ayurvedic *panchakarma* treatments for cervical spondylosis. *Nasya* helps reduce neck tension and inflammation, while *vasti* balances

vata dosha, relieving stiffness and pain. Together with tailored workouts and nutritional guidance, these treatments aim to improve neck mobility and overall spinal health.

- Cervical spondylosis, similar to *greeva stambha*, is a *vata dosha* imbalance, affecting the *vyana vayu* that governs movement. Common symptoms include headaches, neck pain, tingling, and vertigo. Ayurveda offers treatments such as *nadi sweda* (local heat) and *vatahara* therapies to reduce inflammation and muscle spasms, alongside Ayurvedic medications and *panchakarma* therapies to help manage the condition and improve overall healing.
- *Greeva stambha* (cervical spondylosis) is treated by addressing *vata dosha* imbalances with *vata*-suppressing therapies such as local application of *vatahara taila*, *nadi sweda* (local steam), and *guggulu*. These treatments use *snehana* (oil massage) and *swedana* (hot fomentation) to counteract the cold and rough properties of *vata*, reduce stiffness and pain, and improve mobility.
- *Vatahara* treatment in Ayurveda – using *guggulu* preparation, *vatahara taila* (topically), and steam with *vata*-suppressing decoctions – helps treat cervical spondylosis (*greeva stambha*) by reducing inflammation and muscle spasms. This improves blood circulation and nerve function in the affected area, leading to clinical relief and better overall function.

Chapter 6

ARTHRITIS

Arthritis, or joint pains, may grip the body at any age, and essentially interferes with everyday living, including simple activities like moving, exercising and merely managing your own self. Not only at the physical level, this particular disease also affects mental health, as well as influences emotional grounds. The common lab tests undertaken for confirming various types of joint diseases are X-ray of the joint, MRI scan, RA factor, uric acid, ESR, calcium, etc.

Disease Introduction

Arthritis refers to the health condition of joint disease that causes inflammation, soreness, swelling, as well as stiffness. Largely, it is apparent in conditions of osteoarthritis, rheumatoid arthritis and gouty arthritis or gout. Arthritis is disabling for the individual.

Signs and Symptoms

- Tenderness and painful joints with limitation of movements.

According to Ayurveda, stress, early aging, sluggish metabolism and poor nutrition, as well as lifestyle, all contribute to excessive *vata* and *ama* and, eventually, lays the foundation of the disease of arthritis. The subsistence of too much *vata* in the joints, which dries out the bone and cartilage tissues, is referred in the ancient healing as causative for this disease. Moreover, Ayurveda states that joint instability and excruciating pain, as experienced in arthritis, can result from an imbalance in the *vata dosha* or the air body humour. It is also evident that inflammation between joints can also result from the fluids in the joints drying up if a person's *vata dosha* increases. This makes it difficult to move around and eventually results in arthritis.

- There is pain in the affected joints, which may amplify on movement but normally decreases with rest.
- ` Stiffness of joints and wasting away of muscles.
- Generally, there is pain and inflammation in multiple joints, along with inflexibility and symmetrical swelling of peripheral joints.
- Morning stiffness is often experienced.
- The skin may develop subcutaneous fibrous nodules.
- `There is a loss of hunger, general weakness, along with apparent weight loss and progressive deformities of the joints as the disease progresses.

AYURVEDIC UNDERSTANDING OF THE DISEASE

According to Ayurveda, arthritis develops mainly due to accumulated toxic matter, which further results in an imbalance of the three *doshas* – *vata, pitta* and *kapha*.

When the food we eat is not digested properly, it causes *ama* (toxins) which circulates through the entire body and accumulates in the bones and joints causing arthritis. Due to weakness of gastric fire or *agni*, when food remains undigested, this undigested juice (*ama rasa*) intermingles with the vitiated *doshas* or body humours, *vata* (air), *pitta* (fire) and *kapha* (phlegm), and results in the formation of the disease.

Ayurveda specifies that pain and stiffness in the joints results mainly due to imbalance and vitiation in the *vata dosha* (air body humour).

According to Ayurveda, arthritis is categorized into three main types –

1. Osteoarthritis, which is regarded as *sandhigata vata*;
2. Rheumatoid arthritis or *ama vata*; and
3. Gout or gouty arthritis, or *vata rakta*.

Osteoarthritis

Ayurvedic Name: ***Sandhigata Vata***

- There is tenderness and degeneration of the joints with limitation of their movements.
- The affected joints experience pain, which increases on movement but decreases with rest.
- The pain may also increase with changes in weather.

Recommended Herbs and Home Remedies

- Hot paste of fenugreek seeds, or *methi dana,* can be applied locally on the joint for relief.
- The seeds and leaves of papaya are believed to be helpful in decreasing pain and swelling. As for relief, apply

warm papaya leaves as hot fomentation on the affected joints or crush papaya seeds and mix with mustard oil for local massage.

- *Til* (sesame seeds) helps the *vata dosha* to subside, which, when aggravated, results in a number of ailments like muscular and joint pains. *Til* oil may be used for massaging the painful joints.

Rheumatoid Arthritis

Ayurvedic Name: ***Ama Vata***

- Generally, there is poly-arthritis, with pain, stiffness and symmetrical swelling of the peripheral joints.
- The small joints of the fingers and toes are affected first.
- Morning stiffness is experienced.
- Skin may develop subcutaneous fibrous nodules.
- Some other signs are loss of hunger, weakness, weight loss and characteristic deformities of the joints as the disease progresses.
- The R.A. factor is positive in lab tests.

Recommended Herbs and Home Remedies

- Take a pinch of saffron mixed in warm cow's milk at bedtime.
- Use erand oil for massaging the joints. You may also take it in a dose of 20 ml, mixed in hot milk, at bedtime.
- Add camphor to the oil normally used for local massage of the affected joint, e.g. mustard oil, sesame seed oil or any medicated oil. This helps relieve the inflammation, swelling, as well as pain.

- Applying clove oil locally is also beneficial for relieving pain in the malady of arthritis. For this, massage warm clove oil on the site of pain.
- Take *guduchi* or *giloy* in powder form in the dosage of 3–5 grams, twice a day, along with warm water.

Rheumatoid arthritis and *ama vata* have similar characteristics. The primary pathogenic factors that are the basis for *ama vata* (rheumatoid arthritis) are *vata* and *ama*. It is regarded to be a disease with *madhyam rogamarg* (medium-level disease). The primary symptoms like *sandhishool, sandhisotha* and *sandhigraha* (joint pains and swelling) manifest in *asthi* and *sandhi* (bones and joints). According to clinical symptomatology, *ama vata* is equivalent to the condition known as rheumatoid arthritis in contemporary medical literature.

Moreover, being prone to stress, keeping a busy schedule, in addition to poor eating habits, are all contributing factors to a rise in *ama*-related illnesses. *Ama vata* is among the most prevalent diseases.

In the ancient history of medicine, Madhavkar (700 CE) was the first scholar to refer to *ama vata* as a distinct disease in Ayurveda. The morbidity and disease process in *ama vata* are influenced by two factors, *ama* and *vata*. *Ama*, the primary causal factor, is created when the metabolic and digestive systems malfunction. *Vata* results from *vata dosha* aggravation and imbalance. *Ama vata* manifests as pain, stiffness, swelling, soreness and other symptoms when *ama,* with *vata,* becomes localized in the body's tissues and joints.

Gout

Ayurvedic Name: ***Vata Rakta***

- Generally, there is throbbing pain that starts from a single joint and later spreads to other joints.

- The joints are hot, painful and swollen with glossy skin.
- There may be disability and deformity of the joints in chronic cases.
- There is functional and movement loss as the disease progresses.
- In the lab tests, the serum uric acid gets elevated.

Recommended Herbs and Home Remedies

- Take 2–4 flakes of garlic on empty stomach.
- Use ginger for hot fomentation. For this purpose, mix dry ginger powder in sesame oil and massage on the joint.

According to Ayurveda, arthritis is characterized by a progressive deterioration of the joints causing swelling and discomfort. The primary symptoms of arthritis are stiffness and uneasiness in the joints. This makes it difficult to perform basic activities like walking, jogging or even standing. As people age, the issue generally becomes more apparent. Gout and uric acid crystal development can also result from an overabundance of uric acid in the blood. And the kind of Ayurvedic treatment needed for arthritis and joint pains depends on the nature and severity of the ailment.

Herbs that Help

- Use cow's ghee to fry small pieces of ginger and take 2–3 pieces with daily meals.
- Ayurvedic herbs like *alsi*, aloe vera and *giloy* are recommended.
- Pound together condiments like *saunf*, *ajwain* and *methi dana* in equal proportions and take a pinch or two of the mixture with warm water after meals.

- The Ayurvedic herbs *eranda* and *guggul* help in digestion of *ama,* thus relieving tenderness and hardness in the joints.
- Mix dry ginger powder in sesame oil and massage the joints. Follow it up with hot fomentation.
- Prepare a powder by pounding the dried fruit of *harad* and take it in a dose of 3–5 grams, along with warm water, once or twice a day.
- Soak one-fourth to half a teaspoon of fenugreek (*methi dana*) in a glass of water overnight. Take this in the morning, mixed into a teaspoon of honey.
- Pound some fenugreek seeds dried ginger. Take half a teaspoon each of both the powders mixed into some jaggery. This can be taken twice daily.
- Warm sesame oil (*til taila*) or mustard oil (*sarson taila*) and mix into the same powders of turmeric, garlic and some *kapur*. Use this oil for massaging the joints. Cover the area with a warm compress afterwards.
- Soak about half a teaspoon of black *til* seeds in a glass of water overnight. Take this water along with seeds in the morning.
- Chew the leaves of the *harsingar* plant (3–4 leaves), along with warm water, twice a day.

Other Herbs

- Cardamom (Elettaria cardamomum)
- *Kantkari* (Solanum xanthocarpum)
- Clove (Syzygium aromaticum)
- Garlic
- Black pepper
- Grapes (Vitis vinefera)

- Mint (Mentha spicata)
- *Adusa* (Adhatoda vasica)
- *Tulsi* (Ocimum sanctum)
- Asafoetida (Ferula foetida)
- *Mulethi* (Glycyrrhiza glabra)
- *Erand* (Ricinus communis Linn.)
- *Methi dana* (Trigonella foenum)
- *Amba haldi* (Curcuma amada)

According to Ayurveda, *vata dosha* has a major impact on joint stiffness and other discomforts associated with arthritis because it is linked with mobility. An imbalance in *vata* can affect the nutrition of the tissues, while lowering the amount of lubricants that shield the joints and even result in stiffness and pain when moving.

Turmeric's potent anti-inflammatory qualities may help reduce joint stiffness and pain associated with osteoarthritis. Additionally, the herb *ashwagandha* helps to reduce inflammation and improve joint mobility. Additionally, *guggulu* reduces inflammation and improves joint mobility. Ayurvedic treatments for arthritis may involve taking Ayurvedic medicine, herbals, dietary changes and exercise.

Recommended Home Remedies

- Heat a bag of sand and use as a hot compress over the painful and swollen joints.
- *Sarson taila* may be used extensively to massage the joints as this provides strength and warmth to the joints as well as muscles. It provides pain relief and acts as a rubefacient for relieving muscular pain and stiffness.
- Apply a hot paste of onion on the site.

- *Til* seeds help to reduce the *vata dosha* or air body humour.
- Drink hot milk with half a teaspoon turmeric added to it (preferably).
- Mix some turmeric powder into aloe vera pulp and heat it on fire. This may be applied to the affected part for relief.
- Garlic juice, when warmed and massaged on the joint, provides relief from pain as well as swelling.

Diet and Lifestyle Management Tips

- It is essential to maintain the right stance and posture.
- Some yoga asanas like *Siddhasana, Vajrasana, Gaumukh Asana, Bhujang Asana,* etc and *pranayamas,* or deep breathing techniques, like *Bhastrika, Nadi-shodhana and Surya-bhedi,* as well as mild exercises help.
- Ayurveda recommends that the diet should contain less of *vata*-increasing foods like rough, light and cold foods. It also forbids eating less or fasting for long periods.
- Avoid staying awake at night and mental stress.
- In case of joint pain, take care of your body weight.
- Most importantly, Ayurveda recommends proper care and avoidance of *vata*-promoting factors in diet as well as lifestyle (*ahara* and *vihara*), which may cause pain and inflammation in the joints, thereby resulting in arthritis.

Classical Ayurvedic Drugs

- *Dashmoola haritaki*
- *Jirakaadi modak*
- *Rasonpinda*
- *Tamra bhasm*

- *Ajmodadi churan*
- *Panchsam churan*
- *Nimbaadi churan*
- *Vaishvanara churan*
- *Maharasnaadi quath churan*
- *Rasnadi quath churan*
- *Ajmodaadi churan*
- *Amrita ghrit*
- *Pancasama churan*
- *Vyoshaadi guggul*
- *Simhnad guggul*
- *Trayodashang guggul*
- *Vatari guggul*
- *Yograj guggul*
- *Lauh guggul*
- *Amrita guggul*
- *Mahayograj guggul*
- *Rasa parpati*
- *Brihat vatchintamani rasa*
- *Makardwaj rasa*
- *Bangeshwara rasa*
- *Tripurbhairav rasa*
- *Anand bhairav rasa*
- *Brihat vatgajankush rasa*
- *Maha laxmivilas rasa*
- *Mall sindur*
- *Swarnabhupati rasa*
- *Brihat vatgajendra rasa*
- *Sarvavyaadi haran rasa*
- *Brihat Saindhavaadi taila* (Local application)
- *Maha narayan taila* (Local application)

- *Vishgarbha taila* (Local application)
- *Kottamcukkadi taila* (Local application)
- *Maha rasnadi quath*
- *Panchtikta guggul ghrit*
- *Ashoka ghrit*
- *Lakshaadi guggul*
- *Trayodashang guggul*
- *Vatari guggul*
- *Yograj guggul*
- *Mahayograj guggul*
- *Trifla guggul*
- *Ekangveer rasa*
- *Laghu vishgarbha taila* (Local application)
- *Narayan taila* (Local application)
- *Vishgarbha taila* (Local application)
- *Prabhanjana vimardana taila* (Local application)
- *Prasarini taila* (Local application)
- *Maha rasnadi quath*
- *Ajmodaadi churan*
- *Trayodashang guggul*
- *Vatari guggul*
- *Lauh guggul*
- *Vatari rasa*
- *Brihatmashadi taila* (Local application)
- *Prasarni taila* (Local application)
- *Prabhanjana vimardana taila* (Local application)
- *Trifla guggul*

Panchakarma

In Ayurveda, *panchakarma* treatment for arthritis mostly incorporates *vasti* (medicated enemas). In order to balance the *vata dosha*, which is frequently aggravated and vitiated in case of arthritis, *vasti* is a very successful treatment. This *panchakarma* therapy aids in lowering stiffness, irritation and pain in the joints. *Vasti* uses therapeutic oils and herbal decoctions to nourish the tissues and increase range of motion. Personalized nutrition and lifestyle suggestions complement *vasti* to maximize therapeutic effects and support overall joint health.

Some Ayurvedic facts on Arthritis:

1. In the context of arthritis, imbalanced *vata* leads to stiffness, cracking joints and heightened pain. As a result, the joints and connective tissues can be damaged by arthritis, which is a chronic, systemic inflammatory disease. Dryness, coldness and irregular mobility are all signs of an exacerbated *vata dosha*.

    - Rheumatoid arthritis (RA) is referred to as *ama vata*. Ayurvedic medicines, yoga or physical exercise, dietary adjustments and herbal supplements, which are all possible components of Ayurvedic treatment, are recommended for RA management. For arthritis, Ayurvedic treatments include lifestyle alteration, massage therapy, herbal medication and workouts to manage the symptoms.

2. According to Ayurveda, the bones and joints are a site of *vata* in the body, which means that they are prone to *vata* imbalances and have a general affinity for *vata dosha*. The fact that there is a lot of empty space in the

joints themselves, which also correlates with *vata* or air, serves further emphasizes this reality.

- A degenerative joint disease, osteoarthritis (OA) is considered to emerge due to the breakdown of the movable and synovial-lined joint. When it comes to the basic etiology, patho-physiology and clinical characteristics, osteoarthritis falls under the inflammatory category, which is nearly the same as the sandhigata *vata* described in Ayurveda.
- It is advised to reduce the intake of foods that are bitter, astringent and pungent as they make the body feel rougher and drier. More sweet, salty and sour tastes are recommended. *Vata*-pacifying diet also includes the healthful foods like grains, such as quinoa, rye and amaranth, cooked in water with a small amount of ghee (clarified butter).

3. According to Ayurveda, *sandhigata vata*, one of the *vata vyadhis*, is characterized by symptoms like *sandhi-shoola* (joint soreness) and *sandhi-shotha* (joint swelling). Osteoarthritis (OA), a degenerative joint disease, is characterized by the degradation of the moveable and synovial-lined joints. In terms of genesis, patho-physiology and clinical aspects, OA of the joint is addressed in relation to the inflammatory type of joint pains, which is nearly equivalent to the *sandhigata vata* as stated in Ayurveda.

   - Correspondingly, another form of arthritis that Ayurveda refers to is rheumatoid arthritis (RA) or *ama vata*. According to the *madhava nidana* principles of Ayurveda, digestive disorders and inflammatory chemicals are the causes of rheumatoid arthritis.

- Nonetheless, ashtanga hridaya specifies that rheumatoid arthritis is caused by deprived dietary and lifestyle choices that tend to cause inflammation in the body.
- However, both the Ayurvedic approaches described in different texts and by various Ayurvedic acharyas use dietary changes, exercise, herbal supplements and botanicals to help reduce the symptoms of RA.

4. Arthritis is generally referred to as *sandhivata*. The symptoms of this disease include, by and large, joint discomfort, redness, swelling, oedema and inflammation as primary characteristics. On the other hand, arthritis results in inflammation or cartilage tears, which causes the bones to rub against one another. This produces excruciating pain and joint mobility issues. According to Ayurveda, in case of *ama vata*, which is a form of rheumatoid arthritis, the symptoms include: *angamarda*, or body ache; *aruchi*, or tastelessness; *trishna*, or excessive thirst; *alasya*, or lethargy; *gourava*, or heaviness in the body; *jwara*, or feverishness; early-morning joint stiffness; joint pains (like that of a scorpion sting); and some other signs like constipation, indigestion, fullness in the abdomen and insomnia.
5. In order to lower the aggravated *vata* levels, Ayurveda recommends specific treatments for joint strengthening and lubrication. The goal is to repair damaged cartilage and stop additional joint degradation. Ayurveda

treats osteoarthritis and other ailments of joint pains by combining herbals and home remedies, dietary adjustments and lifestyle changes, along with the recommended Ayurvedic medicines. Ayurveda offers a comprehensive strategy for managing osteoarthritis, emphasizing on *dosha* balance restoration and joint health enhancement. Using Ayurveda as an alternative form of treatment can help those suffering from arthritis to move more freely and reduce pain.

6. Rheumatoid arthritis (*ama vata*) and osteoarthritis (*sandhigata vata*) are the two fundamental forms of arthritis described in ancient Ayurvedic text.

   - Within the realm of Ayurvedic medicine, osteoarthritis is classified as a malnutrition disease, which typically affects the body's most susceptible joints. These joints may be vulnerable for a number of reasons including prior infections, trauma or birth defects. Yet, to determine the underlying cause of osteoarthritis, digestive processes or the *agni* (metabolism) is considered, as is the case with other ailments treated by Ayurveda.
   - On the other hand, when the body's *agni*, or digestive fire, as it is known in Ayurveda, is not working correctly, our bodies create waste products and poisons called *ama* in the place of the nutrients that are needed to support the tissues. At the same time, the *vata* or the air body humour builds up in the colon. Toxins (also known as *ama*) generate in the gut, resulting in the emergence of rheumatoid arthritis or *ama vata* disease.

KEY TAKEAWAYS:

- The key takeaway is that, according to Ayurveda, stress, poor nutrition, sluggish metabolism, and lifestyle contribute to excessive *vata* and *ama*, leading to arthritis. The disease is caused by too much *vata* in the joints, which dries out bone and cartilage tissues, causing joint instability, pain, and inflammation.
- In Ayurveda, arthritis is believed to develop primarily due to accumulated toxins (*ama*), which result in an imbalance of the three *doshas* – *vata*, *pitta* and *kapha*. When food is not properly digested, *ama* (undigested food matter) circulates through the body and accumulates in the bones and joints, leading to arthritis. The weakened gastric fire (*agni*) causes undigested food (*ama rasa*) to combine with vitiated *doshas*, leading to the disease. Pain and stiffness in the joints are primarily attributed to vitiated *vata dosha*.
- Osteoarthritis (*sandhigata vata*) in Ayurveda is caused by *vata dosha* imbalance, leading to joint tenderness, pain that worsens with movement and weather changes, and limited mobility.
- Rheumatoid Arthritis (*ama vata*) in Ayurveda involves polyarthritis with pain, stiffness, and swelling of peripheral joints, particularly in fingers and toes. It includes morning stiffness, possible skin nodules, and systemic signs like weakness, weight loss, and joint deformities.
- Gout (*vata rakta*) in Ayurveda is characterized by throbbing pain in one joint, spreading to others. Affected joints are hot, swollen, and painful with glossy skin.

Chronic cases may lead to joint deformity, functional loss, and elevated serum uric acid levels.

- In Ayurveda, arthritis is marked by joint deterioration, swelling, and discomfort, leading to stiffness and difficulty with movement. With age, the condition worsens, and excess uric acid can cause gout. Ayurvedic treatment for arthritis depends on the specific nature and severity of the condition.
- In Ayurveda, arthritis is referred to as *sandhivata* and is characterized by joint discomfort, swelling, and inflammation. For *ama vata* (rheumatoid arthritis), symptoms include body ache, lack of appetite, excessive thirst, lethargy, joint stiffness, scorpion-like pain, and digestive issues such as constipation and indigestion.

Chapter 7

DEPRESSION

Depression is a disease of the mind which tends to intensify a number of psychological and neurological diseases.

SIGNS AND SYMPTOMS

- Lack of interest in small delights and obvious mood changes.
- Feeling of misery, hopelessness, horrifying thoughts, restlessness and loss of sleep.
- Habitual mindset of sadness, lassitude, despair and bad temper.
- General weakness and frequent fatigue.
- Impairment of digestion, constipation and decreased hunger.
- Experiences of anxiety and memory loss.
- Gloomy mood, low confidence and lack of enthusiasm and general interest.
- Suicidal attempts or repeated thoughts of death in case of severe depression.

- Social withdrawal.
- Low or complete absence of appetite, accompanied by apparent weight loss.

In Ayurveda, mental imbalances are considered a significant factor in the development of depression and other psychological conditions. According to this perspective accumulation of chronic fatigue may give rise to greed. This unchecked greed is believed to foster cruelty, which in turn may result in dishonesty. As these imbalances escalate, they can manifest as intense emotions such as passion, rage, vanity, hatred, and fear, ultimately leading to sadness, grief, anxiety, depression and other mental disturbances. Acharya Charaka emphasizes that the root cause of psychiatric disorders is the improper application of the mind. Overthinking is seen as a major mental burden, and when the mind is misused or overwhelmed, it can lead to mental instability. Conversely, when the mind is utilized in a balanced and conscious manner, it promotes mental well-being and emotional stability. Thus, Ayurveda encourages the mindful and appropriate use of mental faculties to maintain optimal mental health.

Ayurvedic Understanding of the Disease

Vishado Rogavardhanam

This means that the mental state is the principal factor that may cause for worsening of the condition of any disease.

This disease is mainly termed as *avsada.* Although *vishada* and *avasada* are the two conditions that are recognized as depression in Ayurveda, the basis of this disease is imbalance or vitiation of the three *doshas* viz. *vata, pitta* and *kapha* or the air, fire and phlegm body humours, as well as a discrepancy in the mental states of *rajas* and *tamas*.

Ayurveda believes that the human body as well as the mind is ruled over by the three *doshas*. When these are in a balanced state, they endorse healthiness of the body and mind. However, vitiation of any of the three *doshas* results a disease both in the bodily as well as psychic spheres. Moreover, as stress (physical and mental) interferes with the natural balance of the *doshas*, the body loses its natural wellness and depression sets in. Further, there is an increase and imbalance in the mental states of *iccha* (desire) and *dwesh* (repulsion), largely triggered by stress and strain.

When the mind is affected, Ayurveda specifies that:

- Vitiation in the *vata dosha* (air) destroys mental sense and gives rise to grief and infatuation.
- When the *pitta* (fire) manifests and increases, it produces excessive fear, lust and grief.
- Imbalances in the *kapha* (phlegm) cause lethargy, anxiety and indiscrimination.

According to Lord Punarvasu Atreya, the root cause of mental conditions like depression is *pragyapradha*, or intellectual blasphemy. The patient disregards the deity, ascetics, ancestors, *gandharvas, yaksas, raksasas, pisachas,* preceptors, elders, adepts, teachers and other revered people because of this cerebral blasphemy. Also, he engages in unwanted and other inauspicious behaviours. Ayurveda recognizes three mental humours (*satva, rajas* and *tamas*) and three bodily humours (*vata, pitta* and *kapha*). According to Acharya Charaka, the *gunas* are *satva* (peace, balance and stability), *rajas* (momentum, desires and anticipation), and *tamas* (*gloom* and inertia). According to Charaka, *satva* is the normal state of a stable mind, but the prominence or imbalance of the other two mind humours (*raja* and *tama*) is the origin of many psychiatric problems. This eventually leads to the disease of depression.

Herbs that Help

- *Brahmi* (Bacopa monneri)
- *Gulkanda* (Rose jelly)
- *Kushmanda* (Benincasa hispida)
- *Shankhapushpi* (Convulvulus pluricaulis)
- *Jatamamsi* (Nardostachys jatamansi)
- *Khas* (Vetiveria zizanoides)
- *Chandan* (Sandalwood)
- *Vacha* (Acorus calamus)
- *Ashwagandha* (Withania somnifera)

Recommended Home Remedies

- Mix one teaspoon of asparagus powder with half a spoon of honey. Take this twice daily, along with warm cow's milk.
- Peel almonds (soaked overnight) and take them in the morning, chewing slowly. Add to this half a teaspoon of *mishri* (crystalline sugar) and a pinch or two of black pepper powder.
- Regular intake of honey helps to fight the feeling of depression. Include this in your daily diet.
- Drink *amla* juice, about 20 ml, once or twice a day.
- Shallow fry a few *Brahmi* leaves in desi ghee. To this, add pounded black pepper powder and some sugar. This may be taken once or twice daily.

- Add honey and a few drops of almond oil to a powder *brahmi* and *shankhpushpi* (Ayurvedic herbs). Take this regularly (3–5 grams) with milk.
- Boil the husk of one teaspoon of dry coriander in a glass of milk. Take this with half a teaspoon of *mishri*, preferably at bedtime.
- Dry *bramhi* in shade. Pound it into a powder. Take one teaspoon, with milk, once or twice a day.
- Drink aloe vera juice in the dosage of 20 ml twice a day.
- Add a pinch of saffron to milk and take it, preferably at night, before going to sleep.
- Crush some white gourd (*safed petha*). Drink the extracted juice in a dose of 20–30 ml twice a day.

In Ayurveda, MDD (major depressive disorder) may be closely associated with *vishada* and *avasada* in mild cases and *kaphaja unmada* in severe cases. *Vishada* is listed as one of the *vataja natatmaja vikaras* in Ayurvedic scriptures. *Vishada* is more common in *heena satwa purusha* (individual with decreased mental strength), according to *Charaka Samhita*. *Avasada* (derangement) of the *manas* (thought), *vaak* (speech) and *kaya* (body) are among the indications. Coexisting medical disorders are made worse by *vishada*. According to *kaphaja unmada*, Ayurveda offers good remedies for depression. *Vataja unmada chikitsa* is also included in *vataja* manifestations. *Snehapana, snidga virechana, sarvanga bahyanga* and *mastiskya chikitsa* may be helpful. Combining *panchakarma* with oral drugs, *satwawajaya and daiwivyapashraya* play an important role in the comprehensive management of MDD.

Classical Ayurvedic Drugs

- *Kushmand ghrita*

- *Balarishta*
- *Sarswatarishta*
- *Chavikasava*
- *Chyavanprash avleha*
- *Vat kulantak rasa*
- *Brahm rasayana*
- *Brihat vat chintamani rasa*
- *Chintamani chaturbhurja rasa*
- *Makardwaj vatti*
- *Bramhi vatti*
- *Ashwagandharishta*
- *Ashwanagandha kshirpaka*
- *Sarswatarishta*
- *Brahmi ghrita*
- *Manasamitra vatakam*
- *Samriti sagar rasa*

Diet and Lifestyle Management Tips

- *Satvik* diet is advised as it enhances positivity of the mind. This requires increased intakes of seasonal fruits, vegetables, sprouts and crops.
- Spicy meals, fried foods and fast food must be avoided. It is always better to refrain from taking highly sugary and maida-based food stuffs.
- Easy to digest meals, which are likable and preferably home-cooked, are suggested.
- Ghee, *mung* (green gram *dal*), cow's milk, wheat and honey are advised on a regular basis.
- Eating more vegetarian foods, along with good amounts of water, also helps.

- Avoid non-vegetarian food, smoking and alcoholic drinks.
- Take a piece of *amla murabba* and/or one teaspoon of *gulkand* (rose jelly), along with warm milk daily.
- Waking up early in the morning and walking in the fresh air help. This is because the ultraviolet rays that are emitted during sunrise work as a mind stimulator as well as mood dilators.
- Meditating for 15–30 minutes every day or simply taking long breaths in silence must be a way of life.
- Practising mild to moderate Yoga poses, like *Shavasana* and *yoga nidra,* in addition to some deep breathing exercises, like *Anulom-Vilom* and *Bhramari pranayamas,* is necessary.
- Laughter therapy and positive thinking is encouraged. Friends and family should consciously avoid negative talk.
- Use aroma oils, such as lavender, in bath, or burn them in the house.
- Massage the soles of the feet with some warm oil, like sesame seed oil. Also, using some cooling oils, like *elaadi tailam* or coconut oil, to massage the scalp daily is recommended.
- Mintain proper hygiene, such as everyday bathing and wearing clean and washed clothes that are comfortable.
- Sleeping for 7 to 8 hours at night is mandatory.
- Ayurveda *panchakarma* therapies of *shirodhara* and *nasya* are recommended. Apply desi ghee or almond drops.
- Consciously connect with all five natural elements i.e. ether, air, sun, water and earth.

- Keep yourself mentally occupied during the day in creative activities that encourage happiness and optimistic thoughts.
- In severe cases of depression, consult a psychiatrist or psychologist.

For relieving depression, Ayurveda recognizes the role of psychosocial stress. The Ayurvedic integrative protocol is helpful in managing *kaphaja unmada* or MDD. This is because it not only helps in decreasing *kapha* and *vata doshas* (biological substrates of depression) and components of *manodusti* (mental instability), but also eventually amplifies *manabala* (mental strength) by restructuring *mana,* or the *mind,* through reworking *chintya, vicharya, uhya, dheya, sankalpa* (various thought processes) and *buddhi* (cognitive restructuring), leading to changes in *bhakti, sheela, chesta* and *achar* (mental processes of positive steadiness of the mind). In the long run, these help in *swasthya* (health promotion) through the balancing of internal milieu (*shareerik* and *manasik dosha* balance or maintaining physical and mental equilibrium) and also the external milieu through social and spiritual well-being

Panchakarma

Shirodhara, nasya and *vasti* are some of the *panchakarma* remedies advised for depression by Ayurveda. *Shirodhara* is the practice of dripping herbal oils onto the forehead to ease tension and promote mental calmness. On the other hand, *nasya* (nasal administration) works by passing medicinal oils through the nasal passages to improve mood and dispel mental fog. Nevertheless, by balancing the *vata dosha, vasti* (medicated enemas) also helps to reduce anxiety and support mental stability. These specific *panchakarma* treatments aid in enhancing mental clarity and emotional well-being when paired with a diet that is supportive, along with lifestyle modifications.

Some Ayurvedic facts on Depression:

1. Known as *shad-ripu* (six foes), six mental illnesses are said to be the primary causes of mental disorders. These are *krodha* (anger or irritability), *lobha* (greed), *moha* (personal over-attachment or likes and dislikes), *mada* (ego or arrogance), *matsa* (jealousy, envy, etc.) and *kama* (wrong or right desires). The most significant and crucial component of *mano-rogas* (mental disease) is kama or unfulfilled desire. In the first chapter of *sharir sthana*, Acharya Charaka states that *upadha* (desire) is the prime cause of distress (both physical and mental disease and disturbance) in the body. This lays the foundation of the disease of depression.
2. Avoiding *upadha* (desires) eliminates all forms of mental and bodily disruption. Acharya Charaka compares upadha to the web of a cob or silkworm. According to him, a silkworm produces suicidal threads for itself. An ignorant individual who is spellbound in material sufferings also provides for his own desires by using a variety of goods. However, a smart person, who avoids sensory stimuli because they are as deadly as a burning fire, does not suffer from the consequences. The bulk of physical and mental illnesses have unmet aspirations as their root cause. According to Acharya Charaka, non-human entities such as demons, gods, ghosts, etc., can enter the body and cause mental illnesses such *dev*

unmada, which are psychological disturbances. These eventually lead to mental diseases like depression.

3. Depression is occasionally mentioned in historical Ayurvedic literature as both an emotional state and a sickness (*manasika vyadhi*). Ayurvedic treatments for depression include *shamana chikitsa*, *vashpa sweda*, *shirodhara* and *sarvang snehan*. When these therapies work together, they ease depression.
4. In order to effectively treat psychiatric problems, Ayurveda provides an integrated strategy that includes *satvavajaya* practices like yoga and counselling, as well as *yukti vyapashraya chikitsa*, which restores *dosha* equilibrium.
5. Along with Ayurvedic medicines, Ayurveda emphasizes yoga, meditation and *panchakarma* procedures for the treatment of depression.
6. Ayurveda believes that the mental states of the *trigunas* – *satva*, *rajas* and *tamas* – are expressed through the manifestation of the mental processes, functions, and consciousness. These *gunas* are in charge of the psychological differences between people, which can be seen in the way they behave, or psychological characteristics.

    - *Bhaya* (fright) and *moha* (delusion) are the main sources of depression, while tamo *guna* is the chief contributing factor. Depression is an illness (*manasika vyadhi*) as well as an emotional condition (*manasika bhava*). The two disorders listed in the Ayurvedic *samhitas*, which closely resemble depression, are *vishada* and *avasaada*.

- Charaka says, *Vishado rogavardhananaam*, which means that depression is the primary cause of worsening of a disease. Among the category of eight *vataja nanatmaja vikaras*, it falls under one, which indicates that depression cannot occur without the involvement of *vata dosha*.

7. Ayurveda describes *vishada* or *avasaada* to be associated with the disease of depression. According to Ayurvedic science, there is correlation between *satva* (mind) and *sharira* (body). Moreover, it has been indicated that both sharira and mana are places of disease manifestation, as well as the maintenance of physical and mental health. *Manasika doshas* (*rajas* and *tamas*) gradually intensify when *sharirika dosha* is disrupted; as a result, mental disease develops in addition to physical illness, and vice versa. It is believed that depression results from a disruption of the body's essential components, including *satva, gyan indriye, karm indriye, rasa dhatu, trigunas, tridosha* and *manovaha srotas.* Not only this, suicidal thoughts could as as a consequence of depression. A positive and healthy mind keeps the body healthy, increases *satva guna* and speeds up the healing of physical ailments. This can be best achieved by an Ayurvedic psychological approach.

Key Takeaways:

- Ayurveda links mental imbalances to the development of psychological conditions like depression. Chronic fatigue, unchecked greed, and escalating emotions like passion, rage, and fear can lead to sadness, grief, and anxiety. Overthinking is seen as a significant burden, and mental stability is achieved by consciously applying the mind in a balanced way. Acharya Charaka emphasizes that proper mental use promotes emotional well-being.

- Lord Punarvasu Atreya attributes the root cause of mental conditions like depression to *pragyapradha* (intellectual blasphemy), which involves disregarding revered individuals and engaging in inauspicious behaviors. Ayurveda recognizes three mental humours – *satva* (balance), *rajas* (desires), and *tamas* (gloom) – with an imbalance in *rajas* and *tamas* leading to mental instability, including depression, as explained by Acharya Charaka.
- In Ayurveda, Major Depressive Disorder (MDD) can be associated with conditions like *vishada* and *avasada* (mild cases) or *kaphaja unmada* (severe cases). These conditions involve imbalances in mental humours, particularly *vata*, and require treatments like *snehapana*, *snidga virechana*, and *panchakarma*. *Satwawajaya* (mental stabilization) and *daiwivyapashraya* (spiritual healing) also play crucial roles in managing depression.
- Ayurveda links depression to imbalances in the *doshas*, particularly *kapha* and *vata*. By integrating mental and physical treatments, such as *panchakarma*, and focusing on mental restructuring, it aims to restore balance and mental strength. The protocol not only addresses biological and psychological factors but also promotes overall health and well-being, both internally and socially.

- In Ayurveda, avoiding *upadha* (desires) is key to preventing mental and physical disturbances. Acharya Charaka compares unfulfilled desires to the destructive threads of a silkworm, symbolizing how unchecked desires lead to suffering. He also highlights that external forces, like demons or spirits, can cause mental illness, including depression, when the mind is overwhelmed by desires. Recognizing and managing these desires is crucial for mental health and well-being.
- In Ayurveda, depression is linked to imbalances in the body's *doshas* and the mind's qualities, particularly when *satva*, the mind's balance, is disrupted. This mental disruption can lead to physical illness and, in severe cases, suicidal thoughts. Ayurvedic treatments aim to restore balance and promote mental well-being for overall health.

Chapter 8

THYROID DISEASE

Thyroid disease is the ailment in which the working of the thyroid gland is impaired (either decreased or increased). Thyroid gland is the master gland for metabolism in the human body. When the thyroid gland is not able to function properly, it adversely affects health. Generally, the thyroid disease ranges in the category of diseases of metabolism and endocrine glands.

There are two basic types of thyroid disease – **Hypothyroidism** and **Hyperthyroidism**. Hypothyroidism is a more common condition in which the thyroid gland does not produce adequate amount of the thyroid hormones, Thyroxine (T4) and Triiodothyronine (T3). Hyperthyroidism is a condition in which the thyroid is overactive and produces the thyroid hormones in excess.

Signs and Symptoms

Hypothyroidism may present a wide variety of symptoms:

- Weight gain without eating enough.
- Anxiety and depression.

- Low energy level.
- Generally, digestion is affected.
- Severe and recurrent constipation and flatulence.
- Acute dryness of skin.
- Parched and brittle hair causing hairfall.
- Joint and muscular pain.
- Women may present symptoms like menorrhagia (heavy and prolonged menstruation) and infertility.
- Oedema and water retention.

In hyperthyroidism, the symptoms are:

- Anxiety.
- Rapid heart rate.
- Unexplained weight loss, despite surplus eating.
- Shallow respiration.
- Strong mental temperament.
- Diarrhoea.
- Heat intolerance.
- Flushing.
- Menstrual disturbance.
- Fatigue.
- Bulging of the eyes.

Ayurvedic Understanding of Thyroid Disease

In Ayurvedic text, thyroid disease is known by the name *gala ganda*, although this name also encompasses the disease goitre.

Ayurveda believes that, in this particular disease, there is aggravation or increase of the *kapha dosha* (phlegm body humour) and decrease of *pitta dosha* (fire body humour). This

Due to the non-specific symptoms and the lack of screening guidelines, hypothyroidism could normally be difficult to detect. Determining when to test for hypothyroidism can be challenging since the patients may exhibit mild symptoms or signs that are rather similar to those of other prevalent illnesses, and there are no clear criteria about who should be tested or when. However, fatigue, weight gain, hair loss, mood swings, dyspepsia, dry, rough skin and cold sensitivity are signs of hypothyroidism. According to *sthaulya chikitsa* in Ayurveda, *rasayana, shaman-aushadhi* and certain *pathya* are useful for relieving thyroid disease.

further causes vitiation of *mansa dhatu* and *medha dhatu* or the muscle and fat body tissues.

Hypothyroidism may be likened to a condition with excessive *kapha* (phlegm) and low *vata* and *pitta* (air and fire). Hyperthyroidism presents itself with excessive *vata* and *pitta doshas*, while there is less or decreased *kapha dosha*.

Herbs that Help

- *Kanchanara*
- *Jatamansi*
- *Shilajit*
- *Ashwagandha*
- *Brahmi*
- *Guggulu*
- *Punarnava*

To be more specific, the herbs recommended by Ayurveda are –

Thyroid issues are viewed in Ayurveda as disruptions in the body's energy pathways and *dosha* (*pitta, kapha* and *vata*) imbalances. The type of thyroid conditions (hypothyroidism and hyperthyroidism), the nature of the imbalance (*vikruti*) and the individual's basic constitution (*prakriti*) can all influence the particular Ayurvedic perspective and remedies for the thyroid disorders. According to Ayurveda, *vata* and *kapha dosha* imbalance is the main cause of hypothyroidism. While *kapha* vitiation can result in congestion, lethargy and weight gain, *vata* imbalance could induce dryness, coldness and decreased metabolic performance.

On the other hand, hyperthyroidism is believed to be a condition where the *pitta dosha* is excessive. Augmented heat, inflammation and extreme metabolic activity can be symptoms of *pitta* imbalance.

Thyroid diseases are thought to be exacerbated by impaired *agni*. *Agni*, the digestive fire that transforms and assimilates nutrients, is highly valued in Ayurveda. Thyroid disorders can result from poor food, lifestyle choices and digestive abnormalities that decrease the *agni*.

Other than this, according to Ayurveda, thyroid issues may be caused by the accumulation of toxins and *ama* (undigested waste). This is because *ama* can obstruct the energy conduits and interfere with the normal functioning of the thyroid gland.

For Hypothyrodism –

- *Kanchanara* (Bauhinia variegata)
- *Ashwagandha* (Withania somnifera)
- *Trifla* (*harad, baheda* and *amla*)
- *Punarnava* (Boerhavia diffusa)
- *Trikatru* (*saunth, kali mirch* and *pippali*)
- *Shilajit*
- *Guggulu*

For Hyperthyroidism –

- *Shatavari* (Asparagus racemosus)
- Aloe vera
- *Guduchi* (Tinospora cordifolia)
- *Neem*
- *Jatamansi* (Nardostachy jatamansi)
- *Brahmi* (Bacopa monnieri)

Recommended Home Remedies

- Boil the bark of the *kachnaar* tree in a glass of water till one-fourth remains. Drink the decoction, thus formed, after filtration, in the dosage of approx. 25 ml twice a day.
- Pound the herb/vegetable, *jala kumbhi* (Pistia stratiotes), to extract the juice. Take 10–20 ml of the juice once a day.
- Ground *jala kumbhi* into a fine paste and apply it on the neck to reduce swelling (in case of goitre).
- Mix one small cup of spinach juice mixed with one teaspoon of cumin seed powder and one teaspoon of honey and take it daily.
- Apply *sasharpaadi lepa* or *sarson taila* (mustard oil) locally.
- Soak one or two teaspoons of dry coriander seeds, overnight. Make a decoction by boiling the seeds in the morning and take it warm.

Classical Ayurvedic Drugs

- *Kanchanar guggul*
- *Punarnava mandoor*

There are two main categories of thyroid gland pathology. Colloidal goitre, abscess and also cancer are examples of structural pathological disorders. Hyperthyroidism and hypothyroidism are examples of functional pathological conditions.

Hormone replacement therapy is used to treat hypothyroidism, a thyroid gland functional pathology that manifests as fatigue, weight gain, hair loss, cold sensitivity, mood swings, dyspepsia and dry, rough skin. This clinical picture must be treated in accordance with *sthaulya chikitsa* since it resembles the state of *sthaulya* or obesity.

The primary emphasis of treatment for this disease is *shodhana* and *shamana*. Many clinical investigations have been conducted on the treatment of hypothyroidism, while *shaman-aushadhis* have proved counteractive and remedial.

- *Yashada bhasm*
- *Kaishor guggul*
- *Ashwagandha arishta*
- *Nityananda rasa*
- *Amritadhaya taila*
- *Mahayogaraj guggul*
- *Punarnava arisht*
- *Shila sindoor vatti*

Diet and Lifestyle Management Tips

- Diet needs to consist of adequate quantities of milk, old rice, barley, green grams, Bengal gram, sugarcane juice, cucumber, etc.
- It is advisable to take lots of raw fruits and vegetables, sprouts, etc.
- Consume less salty and sour foods.

- Increase your water intake considerably. This helps in the process of detoxification.
- Ayurveda encourages a lifestyle that is active, balanced and content.
- Consciously avoid mental stress.
- Having good sleep at night, for about seven to eight hours, is good.
- *Ujjayi* and *Bhramari pranayams, yog nidra* and *Jalandhar bandh* are some effective Yogic activities to pursue.
- Practise meditation and 'OM' chanting every day. This brings about internal support and positivity to overcome thyroid disease.

Panchakarma

Udvartana, *vaman* and *vasti* are among the *panchakarma* remedies for thyroid disorders recommended in Ayurveda. Improved metabolism and thyroid gland stimulation are two benefits of *udvartana*, which is a dry massage using herbal powder. *Vasti* (medicated enema) helps to balance *vata* and enhance endocrine function. Moreover, *vaman* (therapeutic emesis) can balance *kapha dosha* and eliminate toxins. *Virechana*, or purgation therapy, is especially recommended for hyperthyroidism in order to balance *pitta dosha*, detoxify the body and lower excess heat and metabolic activity. The goal of these treatments is to restore thyroid health and balance the vitiated *dosha* in conjunction with dietary and lifestyle changes.

Some Ayurvedic facts on Thyroid disease:

1. *Galaganda* or *gandamala* and *agni vishamyata* are concepts that are broadly mentioned in Ayurveda to address thyroid disease. Numerous etiological elements,

such as *ati sevana* of *madhura rasa* (excess intake of sweet taste in diet), *mithyahara vihar* (incompatible diet and lifestyle) and *vishamasana* (wrong physique gestures), as well as pathogenesis, such as *kaphaja nanatmaja vikara* (multiple ailments relating to *kapha dosha* vitiation), are mentioned in ancient writings. Increased *vata* and *kapha* cause *medo dhatu* (fat tissue) accumulation in the neck region or the *galapradesha*, which, in turn, causes *galaganda*. In order to support the etio-pathogenesis of thyroid disorders in Ayurveda, several Ayurveda classics are used to critically analyse various etiologies and pathogenesis.

2. Thyroid disorders can be taken care of using herb-based remedies and therapies, as mentioned in India's traditional Ayurvedic medical system. According to Ayurvedic principles, the symptoms are generally used to make the diagnosis, which is then confirmed by contemporary laboratory testing. The type of thyroid disease manifestation is taken into consideration when determining the course of treatment. Often, individuals with various thyroid problems, regardless of the gender, respond well to Ayurvedic medicines and herbals like *ksheerabala*, a milk-based preparation of Sida cordifolia.
3. Ayurvedic therapies for thyroid conditions frequently calls for dietary and lifestyle changes. This necessitates eating foods like cooked vegetables, whole grains and nutritional herbs that promote balancing the thyroid gland. Additionally, Ayurveda emphasizes recommended diets and herbals, daily routine upholding, strain reduction strategies and regular exercise routine.

- To promote thyroid health, Ayurvedic herbal remedies should be used frequently. Herbs such as *ashwagandha*, *guggulu*, *brahmi* and *shilajit* benefit the thyroid. It is believed that these herbs increase general well-being, enhance metabolic function and assist in balancing the *doshas*.
- In some circumstances, Ayurvedic *panchakarma*, which are thorough detoxification and rejuvenation techniques, help to get rid of toxins, balance the *doshas* and improve metabolism and general health.

4. Hyperthyroidism is called *ati karshya* mentioned in Ayurveda, which proposes a number of reasons for thyroid malfunction, such as excessive intake of dehydrating foods and drinks (*ruksha annapana*) and extended fasting (*langhana*).

   - It has been demonstrated that *panchakarma* and external treatments like *vamana*, *shirodhara*, *virechana*, *basti*, *udwarthana* and *kashaya seka* are beneficial in treating the symptoms of thyroid disease. Moreover, certain activities like asanas and pranayamas are useful for the thyroid.
   - Some of the Ayurvedic herbs that can aid in relieving the thyroid disease include *kanchnar* or *Bauhinia variegata* (purple mountain ebony), *jatamansi*, *brahm*i, *guggulu*, *shilajit*, *gokshura* and *punarnava*.

5. Rebalancing the body's *doshas* and getting rid of *ama*, or disease-causing toxin, are the main objectives of the Ayurvedic treatment of thyroid disorders. Herbs like

kanchnar guggul, shatavari and herbal formulations like *arogyavardhini vati, chitrakadi vati* and others are part of the Ayurvedic treatment.

- In case of hyperthyroidism, avoiding tough exercise routines and, instead, taking up low-intensity activities may be helpful. Examples of these activities include yoga, tai chi and walking. Thyroid disease is believed to result from a serious imbalance between the *vata* and *pitta doshas.* Including enough milk, pure ghee and milk products in daily diet are recommended, along with the consumption of fresh foods, including bananas, and dry fruits like dates and walnuts.

6. Thyroid disease is expressed in Ayurveda as the vitiated state of the three *doshas.* Mainly, five varieties of thyroid disease are acknowledged, induced by *vata, pitta, kapha,* urinary tract infections (which mainly affect women) and the goitre form, which is evident by an obvious swelling of glands in the neck region. An underlying cause of all *dosha*-induced thyroid disease is believed to be a form of improper dietary digestion. Furthermore, excessive physical activity contributes to the physical component of the *vata*-induced disease, while mental agitation and stress contribute to the psychological component. *Pitta dosha,* or the fire body humour, is responsible for hyperthyroidism. On the other hand, *kapha*-induced hypothyroidism is considered to be the goitre variety of thyroid disease.

7. As mentioned in the traditional Ayurvedic books, it is believed that hypothyroidism is associated with abnormalities of the *jatharagni* and *dhatwagni*, as well as imbalanced *doshas* which show up as abnormalities of the *kapha* and *vata doshas* and also in the *rasavaha*, *raktavaha*, *medovaha*, *sukravaha* and *manovaha srotas*.

    - Systemic disease expression is caused by *dosha*-dushya incompatibility in various *dhatus* or the body tissues. Thus, *deepana, pachana, sroto-shodhana* and *kapha-vata shamana* are all part of the therapeutic plan.
    - However, Ayurvedic writings do not discuss hypothyroidism as an illness. It is believed that *agni*, or the gastric fire, is largely responsible for hypothyroidism. At the *dhatu* level, there is less *agni* because of different *hetus* or causes. As a result, the associated *dhatu* (body tissue) functions are also compromised. Consequently, the *dhatus* are damaged, which are grounds for both mental and physical symptoms. Thus, hypothyroidism is primarily a *vata-kapha samsarga* or aggravation condition, where *vata* aggravates and causes the *kapha dushti* by acting as *yogavahi*. All of these pathogenic elements need to be addressed throughout the healing of hypothyroidism, with particular focus on *dosha*, body strength and mental clarity.

Key Takeaways:

- Hypothyroidism can be challenging to diagnose due to its non-specific symptoms that overlap with other conditions. Common signs include fatigue, weight gain, hair loss, mood swings, and sensitivity to cold. Ayurveda suggests using *rasayana*, *shaman-aushadhi* and *pathya* as treatments for thyroid issues.
- In Ayurveda, thyroid disorders are linked to imbalances in *doshas* (*vata*, *pitta* and *kapha*), with hypothyroidism primarily caused by *vata* and *kapha* imbalances. *Vata* leads to dryness and coldness, while *kapha* causes lethargy and weight gain. Hyperthyroidism is associated with excess *pitta*, leading to inflammation and high metabolic activity. Poor *agni*, improper lifestyle and toxin buildup (*ama*) can exacerbate thyroid issues.
- Thyroid gland pathologies are classified into structural disorders, like goitre and cancer, and functional disorders, like hyperthyroidism and hypothyroidism. Hypothyroidism is treated with hormone replacement therapy, but Ayurvedic treatment emphasizes *sthaulya chikitsa*, focusing on *shodhana* (detoxification) and *shamana* (pacification). *Shaman-aushadhis* have shown effectiveness in managing hypothyroidism symptoms, such as fatigue and weight gain.
- Ayurvedic *panchakarma* remedies like *udvartana*, *vaman*, *vasti* and *virechana* help restore thyroid health by balancing *doshas* and eliminating toxins. These treatments support improved metabolism, endocrine function, and detoxification, complementing dietary and lifestyle changes.

- Ayurveda treats thyroid disorders with herb-based remedies, focusing on symptoms for diagnosis and confirmation through lab tests. The type of thyroid issue determines the treatment approach. Herbal medicines like ksheerabala, a milk-based preparation of *Sida cordifolia*, are commonly effective for thyroid problems in both men and women.
- In Ayurveda, thyroid disease is seen as a result of imbalanced *doshas*, with five types linked to *vata*, *pitta*, *kapha*, urinary tract infections and goitre. Improper digestion is considered the root cause, while excess physical activity and mental stress contribute to *vata* imbalance. Hyperthyroidism is associated with *pitta dosha*, while hypothyroidism, particularly goitre, is linked to *kapha*.

Chapter 9

URTICARIA

This is an allergic skin disease in which elevated patches form on the skin due to intense and forceful itching, while the skin in the affected areas becomes red and pale.

Signs and Symptoms

- Extreme itching, as well as a burning sensation on the skin.
- Formation of wheels or oedema on the affected skin.
- (In severe conditions) Diffused swelling of the mucous membrane of the mouth as well as the throat, which may lead to respiratory distress.

Ayurvedic Understanding of the Disease

The Ayurvedic name for the disease of urticaria is *sheetpitta*. Ayurveda specifies that the skin allergy of urticaria is caused mainly due to imbalance of all the three *doshas* or body humours, viz. *vata, pitta* and *kapha* (air, fire and phlegm). More specifically, an aggravation of *vata* and *kapha doshas,* along

Ayurveda defines *sheetpitta* or the disease of urticaria as *tridoshaj vyadhi* (disease with vitiation of all the three *doshas* viz. *vata, pitta* and *kapha*. However, the main *dushyas* are *rasa* and *rakta* (juice and blood body tissues), while the prominent *doshas* are *vata* and *kapha*. Thus, Ayurveda refers *sheetpitta* as one of the prominent *twaka vikara* (skin disease).

Two *doshas, vata* and *kapha,* are mainly disturbed, and yet *pitta dosha* is also linked to them, resulting in *tridosha prakopa* (imbalance of all the three *doshas*), which causes skin redness, swelling, itching, etc. Reddish patches and skin irritation are the main signs of *sheetpitta*, with moderate to extreme itching of the affected region. In Ayurveda, *shodhana* and *shamana chikitsa* are used to treat *sheetpitta*.

with vitiation of the *pitta dosha* is believed to be responsible for the disease.

According to Ayurveda, urticaria is caused mainly due to incompatible diet intake. As a result, all three *doshas* or body humours are believed to become imbalanced or vitiated.

Ayurveda believes that, in the case of urticarial:

- *Kapha dosha* aggravation causes itching of the skin.
- Burning sensation and sometimes fever and nausea are generally due to *pitta dosha* vitiation.
- Imbalance of and increase in *vata dosha* cause pain.

Herbs that Help

- *Haridra* (Curcuma longa)
- *Neem* bark (Azadirachta indica)
- Mustard oil and rock Salt (local application)
- *Ajwain* (Carom seeds/Bishop's weed)

In Ayurveda, urticarial, or *sheetpitta* is a disorder characterized by red skin rashes, itching and occasional discomfort. In certain instances, there is heat, swelling and a burning feeling. This is an allergic reaction, which is primarily brought on by certain meals. Based on the symptoms, urticaria can be mild, moderate or severe.

Urticaria is brought on by an excess of *sheeta* (cold) over *pitta*, or, to put it in another way, the dominance of the *vata dosha*. Excessive consumption of spicy or salty foods, even excessive dieting and frequently staying awake at night can aggravate *vata*.

Urticaria can be correlated with *sheetapitta,* which is a *tridoshaja vyadhi*. This disease is defined as the eruption of circumscribed oedematous and frequently itchy swellings of the dermis. As per Ayurveda, urticaria can be correlated with *sheetapitta* in terms of clinical features, causative factors and pathogenesis.

- *Giloy/guduchi* (Tinospora cordifolia)
- *Trifla* (*harad, baheda* and *amla*)
- *Munakka* or *kishmish*

Recommended Home Remedies

- Local application of coconut oil or mustard oil may provide relief from itching.
- Taking raw turmeric with milk or water proves useful. It is advisable to take 1–3 grams of this, once or twice a day.
- Massaging with soda bicarbonate along with *saindhav lavan,* added to *sarson taila* (mustard oil) helps relieve the itch.

- In half a bowl of sour curd, add about two teaspoons of mustard oil and juice of one-fourth lemon. Apply this mixture on the affected body parts 5–10 minutes prior to bath. This helps to relieve skin rash and itching.
- Take aniseed or black pepper powder with a glass of warm water twice a day.
    - Purified *shudh geirak* (1 gram), mixed in half a teaspoon honey may be taken once or twice.
    - Mix ajwain and *gur* (jaggery) in the ratio of 1 gram and 2 grams each. This mixture may be taken once or twice a day along with warm water or warm milk.

Classical Ayurvedic Drugs

- *Sarivadyarishta*
- *Sarivadyasav*
- *Brihat manjishthaadi quath*
- *Haridra khand*
- *Kushtha lep*
- *Gandhak yoga*
- *Panna bhasm*
- *Aragvadhaadi quath churan*
- *Kasisaadi ghrit*
- *Rasottamaadi lepa churan*
- *Gandhak rasayana*
- *Pranavallabha rasa*
- *Udaybhaskar rasa*
- *Brihat Somraji taila*
- *Somraji taila*
- *Nilikadya taila*
- *Chandabala lakshaadi taila*

- *Kandunashak taila*
- *Maha marichyaadi taila*
- *Hingulaadi lepa*
- *Kamdudha rasa*
- *Soot shekhar rasa*
- *Marichyaadi taila*
- *Arogya vardhani vatti*
- *Rason kalpa*
- *Vardhmaan pippali kalpa*
- *Triflaadi gutika*
- *Kamdudha rasa*
- *Mahatikta ghrit*
- *Sarsaparilla*

According to *nidaan sevana* (the etiological factor), *sheetpitta* is a *tridoshaja vyadhi,* characterized by the vitiation of *kapha* and *vata doshas* that mix with *pitta* to disseminate throughout the body, both internally and externally.

Internally spreading *tridoshas* result in *dushti* (pathogenesis) of *rasa* and *rakta dhatus*, and their *dushti* or imbalance manifests as symptoms like *varati damstavat sotha* (rash and swelling), *kandu* (itching), *shool* (pain) and *daha* (burning sensation), which are brought on by *pitta, kapha* and *vata*, respectively, and extend to *twaka* or the skin.

All of these symptoms are associated with the disease of urticaria, which is characterized by red, elevated, itchy patches and rashes brought on by the allergens.

Diet and Lifestyle Management Tips

- It is essential to do away with the underlying cause of the disease, if it can be discovered.

- Urticaria skin allergy generally appears due to incompatible diet. In this case, diet correction is the key to combating the skin allergy. Some of the foods or food combinations cause toxicity due to them being conflicting by nature. This incompatible diet is called virudh aahara in Ayurveda and is believed to be the root cause of urticaria or skin allergy.
- Ayurveda cautions against incompatible diet because it creates an impurity in the bloodstream.
- The diet needs to be light and easily digestible. It should include food items like mung dal, old rice, coconut, black grams, petha and warm water.
- Sour and heavy to digest foods must be avoided.
- Eating foods with both hot and cold potency would generate toxicity or *ama*.
- Diet should be compatible with the prevailing climate. For example, eating food that causes warmth in the body during summer may cause more harm than good. Dry fruits, which are generally considered healthy, if overconsumed during summer may affect the body inversely.
- Avoid heavy meals if you have weak digestion.
- Incompatible diet due to natural discrepancy, such as taking fish with milk, must be avoided.
- Sometimes, incompatible diet is repulsive and rather contrary to the basic innate body constitution. This happens when a person with a particular constitution takes more of the diet, which further aggravates the *dosha*. For example, skin allergy manifests easily when a person with increased *pitta*, or the fire humour, keeps on eating hot, fried and spicy food.

- Some food items become incompatible when taken after eating something. For instance, taking cold water after eating ghee is considered incompatible and renders toxicity.
- Ayurveda restricts some diet items like foods with a sour taste, fried, potent, spicy diet and those which are heavy to digest.
- Sometimes, the disease of urticaria is caused by contact with a substance towards which one is more sensitive. This may result in producing a toxic reaction in the blood.
- Drinking hot water, as well using hot water, for bathing is advised.
- Sometimes, it is necessary to take an anti-allergic drug according to the severity of the symptoms.
- In case urticaria persists for a longer time, it is advisable to get your stool tested to rule out any worm infestation. Also in case of chronic ailment with recurrent symptoms, go in for blood tests for skin allergy detection.
- When the toxic overload (*ama* accumulation) is too much to be controlled by diet and lifestyle modifications, herbs and herbals, or home remedies, expelling the toxins by *panchakarma* detoxification might help. Ayurveda sages have mentioned as follows: the diseases managed by diet and lifestyle modifications might sometimes recur; however, those tackled by *panchakarma* usually do not reappear.
- Among the *panchakarma* procedures, *vamana* (therapeutic emesis) and *virechana* (therapeutic purgation) prove to be of significant assistance.

- Being specialized procedures, *panchakarma* should be taken under the close supervision of an Ayurvedic physician.

Panchakarma

Vaman and *vasti* are two Ayurvedic *panchakarma* remedies for severe urticaria. Removing toxins and balancing *kapha dosha* by *vaman* (therapeutic emesis) helps reduce allergic responses and inflammation of the skin. Additionally, urticaria symptoms can be reduced with *vasti* (medicated enemas), which balances the *vata dosha* and aids in the removal of toxins from deep inside the body. With the help of these *panchakarma* therapies, itching and swelling subside as the body is detoxified and *dosha* balance is restored. Personalized food and lifestyle suggestions improve general skin health and help prevent recurrences.

Some Ayurvedic facts on Urticaria

1. Due to the prominence of *kapha* and *vata* in *sheetpitta*, *ushna-tikshna gunatmak kalpa* (drugs and Ayurvedic medications with natural properties of being hot and sharp), such as *laghu sutshekhar rasa*, can be beneficial. *In sheetpitta*, it has been demonstrated that *virechan virechan karma* (purgation), combined with *shaman* (palliative) action is successful in bringing about relief while also nullifying *pitta dosha* vitiation. *Sheeta-amla ahara* (cold and sour tasting food) and *sheeta vihara* (frequent application of coldness in lifestyle) cause the vitiation of *kapha* and *vata doshas* in *sheetpitta*. There is further anubandha or combining of *pitta dosha* with *kapha*. Therefore, it is necessary to break the vitiated

kapha-created *strotavarodha* initially in such a situation. Charaka has recommended *udarda prashamana mahakashya* medications. In addition to removing the *strotavarodha* and normalizing the vitiated *kapha*, *ushna-tikshna-laghu guna* (hot, sharp and light natural properties) and *katu-tikta rasa* (bitter and pungent tastes) help the disintegrated *pitta dosha* to return to its normal state.

2. Ayurveda plays a significant role in offering a thorough remedy for the skin issue of urticaria. Ayurvedic texts mention both the *shamana* (subsisting *doshas* with appropriate internal medicine) and *shodhana* (removing *doshas* from the body by means of applicable *panchakarma* therapeutic techniques). *Shodhana chikitsa* provides improved results with less possibility of recurrence in *bahudosh avastha* (vitiation of multiple *doshas* or body humours) of this condition.

    - In light of this, further drugs have been proposed after the predominance of *rakta*, *pitta* and *vata dosha*. Thus, *irechana is* a fine therapy mentioned in Ayurveda for the disease of urticaria or *sheetpitta*.

3. Since *sheetpitta* is a *tvak vikara* or skin disorder, it can be linked to urticaria. *Sheetpitta* symptoms include itching, burning and pain, as well as wheels or hives that occur all over the body.

    - Ayurvedic treatment for urticaria or *sheetpitta* helps to promptly alleviate the symptoms. In Ayurveda, the word *sheetpitta* is a combination of the terms sheeta, which means cold, and *pitta*, which signifies hot. Therefore, this disease arises when the *sheeta* or coldness tends to predominate the *pitta dosha*, thus causing an imbalance. Just as urticaria is characterized by itchy wheels or lesions that occur unexpectedly on any mucous membrane or area of skin, similalrly, *sheetpitta* is associated with these symptoms and Ayurvedic treatments for *sheetpitta* provide reasonable benefit by Ayurvedic *shodhan chikista* as well as *shaman chikitsa*.

4. Urticaria or *sheetpitta* occurs due to the domination of *sheet* (cold) over the *pitta dosha* or the fire body humour. When a person is exposed to cold weather, *kapha* and *vata doshas* aggravate and eventually combine with the *pitta dosha*. Together, these vitiated *doshas* spread all over the body and create hives on the surface of the skin. As the evident signs and symptoms, *shotha* and *kandu* (swelling and itching), are caused by *kapha dosha* vitiation, *shool* (pain) is caused by *vata dosha* vitiation, while *daha* (burning sensation) is caused by the *pitta dosha*.
5. The three phases of *sheetpitta chikista* mentioned in Ayurveda are *shodhan* for *bahudosha avastha* (involvement of multiple *doshas*), *langhana* with *pachana* for *madhyam dosha avastha* (medium state of *dosha* imbalance) and *langhana* for *alpa dosha* (less *doshas* vitiation).

- *Virechan* and *raktamokshana*, similar to *vamana*, are the best and most efficient treatments in *sheetpitta shodhan* since they help to remove the vitiated *dosha* from the body and prevent recurrence.

- Since *shodhan chikista* helps to clear the clogged *kapha* and *pitta doshas*, it can be regarded as the primary *chikista* (*apunarbhav chikista*).

6. As specified in Ayurveda, the primary causes of *sheetpitta* are the aggravation of *kapha* and *vata doshas* and their combination with the vitiated *pitta dosha*. Thus, *nitya virechan* and *jala dhauti* are believed to soothe the vitiation in the *vata–pitta doshas* and *kapha dosha*, respectively. Also, according to *Charaka Sutra Sthan* (Chapter 16), *sheetpitta* is a condition that is present in *bahudosha avastha* or *lakshana* (signs and symptoms), such as pitaka, kota and *kandu*, and its cure is referred to as *shodhana chikista*, which is dependent on *dosha* dominance. These *shodhana* therapies are mostly used because of their expertise. When *doshas* are aggravated, *shodhana* helps prevent the disease from occurring, which is why *shodhana chikista* is hailed as the first line of treatment. For *shodhana*, *jala dhauti karma* and *nitya virechana* could help to eliminate toxins from the body.
7. Urticaria or *sheetapitta*, as mentioned in Ayurveda, is a *vata*-dominant disorder. The signs and symptoms of *sheetapitta* includes *varati dashta samsthana* that have been described by Acharya Madhavakara. *Chhardi* (vomiting), *jwara* (fever), *vidaha* (burning sensation), *kandu bahula* (severe itching), *toda bahula* (excessive pricking pain) and *shotha* (inflammation similar to an insect bite) are the signs and symptoms mentioned in

Ayurveda. The primary drugs and food items that are used for healing the disease are *sheeta virya* (foods with cold potency), *katu, tikta, madhura, kashaya rasa* (foods containing sweet, pungent, bitter and astringent tastes) and *guru-snigdha guna* (containing the properties of heaviness and oiliness). As a result, they have anti-pruritic, anti-inflammatory, antioxidant and immune-modulatory qualities and function as *tridodhashamaka, rasayana* and *deepana* (invigorate the gastric fire, uphold boosting characteristic and balance all the three vitiated *doshas – vata, pitta* and *kapha.*

Key Takeaways:

- In Ayurveda, *sheetpitta* (urticaria) is considered a *tridoshaj vyadhi*, with *vata* and *kapha* being primarily disturbed, though *pitta* is also involved. It leads to skin redness, swelling, and itching, with the main affected tissues being *rasa* and *rakta*. Treatment includes *shodhana* (cleansing) and *shamana* (palliative) therapies.
- In Ayurveda, urticaria, or *sheetpitta*, is caused by an imbalance of all three *doshas – vata*, *pitta* and *kapha*. Specifically, an aggravation of *vata* and *kapha*, along with *pitta* vitiation, leads to the condition. Incompatible diet intake is considered a primary cause, disrupting the balance of the body humours.
- In Ayurveda, urticaria (*sheetpitta*) is marked by red rashes, itching, and sometimes swelling or a burning sensation. It is caused by an excess of cold (*sheeta sheeta*) over *pitta*, with *vata dosha* dominance. Factors

like consuming spicy or salty foods, excessive dieting, and irregular sleep can aggravate *vata* and trigger the condition. Urticaria is a *tridoshaja vyadhi* and shares clinical features, causes, and pathogenesis with *sheetpitta*.

- In Ayurveda, *sheetpitta* is a *tridoshaja vyadhi*, where the vitiation of *kapha*, *vata* and *pitta doshas* spreads internally and externally. This imbalance affects the *rasa* and *rakta dhatus*, causing symptoms like rash, swelling, itching, pain and a burning sensation. These symptoms are linked to the pathogenesis of urticaria, with red, raised, itchy rashes typically triggered by allergens.
- *Vaman* and *vasti* are effective *panchakarma* treatments for severe urticaria. *Vaman* helps balance *kapha dosha*, reducing allergic reactions and skin inflammation, while *vasti* balances *vata dosha* and detoxifies the body. These therapies, along with personalized diet and lifestyle changes, help relieve symptoms like itching and swelling while promoting overall skin health.
- Urticaria or *sheetpitta* occurs when cold (*sheet*) aggravates *pitta dosha*, leading to a combination of vitiated *vata*, *kapha*, and *pitta doshas*. This imbalance causes symptoms like swelling and itching (*kapha*), pain (*vata*), and a burning sensation (*pitta*) on the skin.

Chapter 10

BRONCHITIS

In this disease, there is inflammation of the bronchial tubes or bronchi of the lungs.

The main symptom of coughing, as is the case in bronchitis, can also be found extensively in some other diseases of the respiratory system. Coughing can be a symptom of bronchial asthma, allergies, TB, pneumonia, COPDs (Chronic Obstructive Pulmonary Diseases) and lung cancers etc.

It must be understood that coughing for at least two months or three consecutive years is largely termed as chronic bronchitis.

Signs and Symptoms

- Mild but irritating cough, mainly allergic cough; dry or unproductive cough, and later on, productive cough with thick, vicious or blood-streaked sputum.
- Discomfort or pain in the chest area.
- Feeling of tightness in the chest.
- Dyspnoea, wheezing sound and fever.
- General malaise and sore throat.

- If signs of cough are ignored or suppressed, it may take the form of a more grave disease like asthma or tuberculosis.

Based on clinical indications and symptoms, the respiratory conditions of bronchitis (*kasa roga*) and asthma (*tamakshwasa*), as mentioned in Ayurveda, can be connected. Numerous causal factors cause both *vata dosha* and *kapha dosha*. When the aggravated *vata dosha* is obstructed by the vitiated *kapha dosha*, it causes irregular movement that manifests as a variety of symptoms, including coughing and dyspnoea, and eventually progresses to the development of bronchitis or *kasa roga*. Herbal formulations, dietary adjustments and lifestyle changes are commonly used in Ayurvedic treatment for bronchitis in order to assist balancing the *doshas* and supporting the body's natural healing processes. Ayurveda also recommends *pranayama,* or deep breathing exercises, and yoga asanas to support the lungs and help alleviate bronchitis symptoms.

Ayurvedic Understanding of the Disease

The Ayurvedic name for the disease of bronchitis is *kasa roga*. Derived from the words *kas ghato*, it implies that when *vata* or the air moves upwards from the throat and head region, it produces a sound of torn-off bamboo bristles.

It is evident that due to the impairment of digestion, an imbalance in all the three *doshas,* or body humours, viz. *vata, pitta* and *kapha*, cause the disease.

There are five main types of bronchitis or *kasa roga* as mentioned in the Ayurvedic texts.

1. Due to the vitiation of *vata dosha* or the air body humour: This principally results in dry cough.

2. Due to the vitiation of *pitta dosha,* or the fire body humour: This causes bleeding and fever, along with cough.
3. Due to the vitiation of *kapha dosha,* or the phlegm body humour: Thist results in productive cough.
4. That which results from an injury or infection.
5. Another type of Bronchitis is caused as a consequence of tuberculosis.

Herbs that Help

- *Tulsi* (Holy basil)
- *Kali mirch* (Black pepper)
- *Pan* leaf (Betel)
- Ginger (Zingiber officinale)
- Turmeric (Curcuma longa)
- *Pippali* (Piper longum)
- *Choti elaychi* (Cardamom)
- Garlic
- *Mulathee* (Liquorice root)
- *Vasa* (Malabar nut)
- *Vacha* (Acorus calamus)
- *Bharangi* (Clerodendron serratum)
- *Talish* (Abies webbiana)
- *Kantakari* (Solanum virginianum)
- *Apamarg* (Achyranthes aspera)
- *Pushkarmool* (Inula racemosa)

Recommended Home Remedies

- Take three grams of turmeric or *haldi* powder once or twice a day, along with warm water.

- Take two to three black peppercorns; add one-fourth teaspoon of cumin seeds and one-fourth teaspoon of rock salt (*saindhav lavan*). Pound and mix the ingredients together and take twice a day, along with warm water.
- Take 2–3 pods of *lavang* or clove, grind them and mix the powder with one teaspoon of honey. Take this twice a day.
- Tea made with fresh leaves of *tulsi* is recommended.
- Mix 5–10 ml of the juice of basil leaves with one teaspoon of honey and take the mixture twice a day to relieve cough and related symptoms of bronchitis.
- Ground together dried ginger or *saunth*, black pepper and long pepper in equal quantities (1–3 grams each) and mix with one teaspoon of honey. This can be taken once or twice a day, depending on the signs and symptoms.
- Cinnamon or *dalchini* powder, along with a pinch or two of powdered black peppercorns and a few drops of ginger juice may be taken twice a day, mixed with a teaspoon of honey.
- Mild massage of *hing* (asafoetida) on the chest helps.
- Mix the juice extracted from betel leaf (5–10 ml approx.) with freshly ground basil, mint and ginger. Add about 4–5 pounded peppercorns to the paste. This preparation can be taken half a teaspoon twice a day, along with a teaspoon of honey.
- It is also advised to gargle with the juice extracted from *pan* or betel leaf.
- Pound 1–2 cardamoms and take the powder mixed into one teaspoon of honey.

- Supplement *tulsi* tea with a pinch each of ground cloves, black pepper and cinnamon. Honey can be added to it in a moderate quantity (when the tea is not hot). This makes it easy to extract phlegm and relieve bronchitis symptoms.

Ayurveda states that poor digestion is the main cause of bronchitis. For this reason, Ayurveda treats the disease with medications that are also used to treat the digestive system and lungs.

According to a reference in ancient Ayurvedic texts, if *kasa* (cough) is present, there must be apparent *vikruti,* or imbalance, of the *kapha dosha,* which can be inferred as a sign of *jihva saamta* (coating of the tongue). The decline in *agni* (gastric fire) and the formation of *saam kapha* are symbolized by *jihva saamta.*

One of the *pranvaha srothodusti janita vyadhi* (disease of the respiratory system) is *kaphaja kasa*, in which the coughing sensation or *kasa vega*, is linked to *bahala ghana nishthivana* (extra thick sputum). The causes and symptoms of chronic bronchitis and *kaphaja kasa* are most closely associated with one another. *Nidana parivarjana* (keeping away from causative factors) is also helpful, along with various forms of *shodana* (purification) and *shamana chikitsa* (curative medications).

Classical Ayurvedic Drugs

- *Sitoplaadi churan*
- *Chyanprash avleha*
- *Vyoshaadi vatti*
- *Talishaadi churan*
- *Rasa sindur*
- *Kaphaghani vatti*

- *Marichyaadi vatti*
- *Rasa parpati*
- *Lavangaadi vatti*
- *Kaphketu rasa*
- *Shring bhasm*
- *Vasavleha*
- *Shringaadi churan*
- *Karpuraadi vatti*
- *Khadiraadi vatti*
- *Chanderamrit rasa*
- *Brihat panchmoolaadi kwath*
- *Mustakaadi avleh*
- *Marichyaadi churan*
- *Agastya haritaki avleh*
- *Kushmand avleh*
- *Praval bhasm*
- *Yav kshar*
- *Praval pishti*
- *Kapha chintamani rasa*
- *Tankan bhasm*
- *Yashad bhasm*
- *Lakshaadi taila (local massage)*
- *Apamarg kshar*
- *Kantakari kshar*

Diet and Lifestyle Management

- Consume less sour foods and fruits.
- Avoid curd.
- Eat less of bananas.
- Avoid damp and cold climatic conditions.
- Keep away from smoking and alcohol.

- Smear the head region with oil. Steam inhalation is also recommended.

PANCHAKARMA

The two *panchakarma* therapies which are effective Ayurvedic treatments for bronchitis are *vaman* and *virechan*. Congestion and mucous can be cleared by *vaman* (therapeutic emesis), which principally removes excess *kapha* from the respiratory tract. On the other hand, *virechan*, also known as purgation therapy, balances the vitiated *pitta dosha*, speeds up metabolism and helps the body detoxify. Together with a tailored diet and lifestyle changes, these therapies aim to naturally enhance lung and respiratory tract function, as well as reduce the symptoms of bronchitis.

As per Ayurvedic texts, bronchitis has a similarity with *kaphaja kasa* (cough due to *kapha dosha*) with respect to *nidanas* (causative factors) like *raja* and *dhuma sevana* (dust and smoke), *vata-kapha prakopaka ahara vihara* (diet and regimen that aggravates *vata* and *kapha doshas*), as well as and *lakshanas* (symptoms) like *kasa* (cough), with *kapha shteevana* (coughing out heavy sputum), *shwasakrichrata* (difficulty breathing), *shukapurnagalasyata* (dry throat) etc.

Management of bronchitis or *kaphaja kasa* requires *samprapti vighatana* (stopping the disease from progressing). This can be accomplished by drugs that provide the natural properties of *agnideepana* (to enhance the digestive fire) and *amapachana* (*detoxification*), and aid *kaphanissarana* (removal of excess mucous).

The ancient Ayurvedic *samhitas* have well-documented respiratory disorders with *kapha* (cough with phlegm) and *shwasa* (breathing difficulty).

Some Ayurvedic facts on Bronchitis:

1. The major symptoms of bronchitis (*kasa roga*) are *kasa* (cough), *kapha stheevana* (expectoration) and *shwasa krichrata* (breathlessness). This disease is included under *prana-vaha sroto-vikaras* (respiratory disorders) and is characterized by chronic cough with expectoration, usually for at least three months in a year and for more than two consecutive years. Often, there are systemic components characterized by impaired nutrition, weight loss and skeletal muscle dysfunction, along with complaints of breathlessness, cough and frequent expectoration. *Agastya haritaki avaleha* is an Ayurvedic formulation that acts as *brimhana* (nutritive or nourishing therapy) and helps to accomplish the *shamana* (healing and decreasing) of *kapha*.
2. According to Acharya Charaka, *kaphaja kasa* is the ultimate result of the *avarana* (covering) of *kapha* to the *gati* (movement) of *prana vayu*. Mucous is produced in chronic bronchitis because of the irritable mucosa of the respiratory tract. Ayurveda believes that the *avarana* of *kapha* to *prana vayu* is the foundation of chronic bronchitis. The *samprapti* or pathogenesis may also be influenced by *agni dushti* (disparity of the gastric fire). Since *avarana samprapti, prana vayu* attains viloma *gati* or the reverse movement of the *vata dosha*. According to Ayurveda, *agni deepana* (invigorating of the gastric fire), *avarana*-hara (removal of the covering), *vata anulomaka* (normal flow of *vata dosha*) and *rasayana* (tonics) should all be incorporated into the therapeutic principle in this disease recovery.

3. Ayurveda treats the root of the problem in order to take care of it. According to the Science of Ayurveda, bronchitis is known as *kasa roga*. Ayurveda states that bronchitis comes about primarily due to impaired and weak digestion and this is the reason why Ayurveda treats bronchitis through drugs that have the ability to restore to health of both the lungs and also of the digestive system.

    - Ayurvedic medicinal formulation of *agastya haritaki avaleha* has *anabhishyandi* (holding on to the oozing out property), *snigdha* (slimy) and *sroto-shodhana* (clearing of the minute channels) and is generally indicated in all types of *kasa* and *shwasa rogas*. Therefore, *agastya haritaki avaleha* is one of the chosen poly-herbal formulations of Ayurvedic medicine for the disease of bronchitis. Initially, the disease may be caused by *vata kopa* (aggravation and vitiation of the *vata dosha*), which would result in *shuska kasa* or dry cough. However, when the disease worsens, *avarana* of *kapha* to pranavayu may occur, which could lead to *sakapha kasa* (productive cough). According to the *Chikitsa Sutra* (treatment treatise) of Ayurveda, *anabhishyandi*, *snigdha* and *srotoshodhana* are useful properties in the drugs. Thus, an Ayurvedic regimen is helpful for treating chronic bronchitis.

4. According to Ayurvedic scriptures, *kasa roga* is a distinct disease or *vyadhi* and a symptom of a number of distressing diseases, each with its own form, symptoms,

indicators, causation, as well as therapy. Critical conditions, including *swasa*, *shosa*, *rajayakshama*, *urakshata*, *rakttapitta*, *granthi* and *arbuda* ailments of the respiratory tract, among others, might develop if *kasa vyadhi* is not treated promptly. *Vataja*, *pittaja*, *kaphaja*, *kshayaja* and *kshataja* are the five varieties of *kasa*. Of these, *kaphaja kasa* is common and, according to its clinical signs, *kaphaja kasa roga*, a disease mentioned in Ayurvedic writings, closely resembles chronic bronchitis.

- According to Ayurveda, *nidanas* (causative factors), such as *raja* and *dhuma sevana* (dust and smoke), *vata-kapha prakopaka ahara vihara* (diet and regimen that aggravate *vata* and *kapha doshas*), as well as *lakshanas* (symptoms), such as *kasa* (cough) with *kapha shteevana* (coughing out mucous from lungs), *shwasa krichrata* (difficult breathing), *shukapurnagalasyata* (dry throat), etc., make bronchitis similar to *kaphaja kasa* (prolonged cough due to *kapha*).
- *Samprapti vighatana*, or impeding the development of the disease, is necessary for the management of *kaphaja kasa*. This can be accomplished with medications that give *kapha nissarana* (elimination of excess mucous), *ama pachana* (detoxification) and *agni deepana* (increasing the digestive fire).
- Two respiratory conditions that relate to the disease of bronchitis and are well-documented in the ancient Ayurvedic *samhita* are *kasa* (cough) and *shwasa* (difficulty in breathing). The main

objective of bronchitis treatment, as per Ayurveda, is balancing the aggravated *vata* and *kapha doshas* by *sanshodhan*, in addition to *shaman chikitsa*, i.e. following detoxification therapies and decreasing excessive *kapha* or phlegm.

5. *Kasa roga*, in Sanskrit, translates to inflammation and obstruction of the lungs, with the defining symptom being *kaphaja kasa*. This means cough that occurs from the vitiated *kapha dosha*, along with aggravated *vata*. Besides these respiratory indications, this disease also results in fatigue and lowered efficiency at home and work, along with signs of hampered digestion, nausea, vomiting and regular headaches.

    - In the management of *kaphaja kasa* (chronic or recurrent muco-purulent bronchitis) , different modes of approach are required at different stages. Adopting a multi-remedies protocol is usually necessary. The most crucial component of treatment is *nidana parivarjana*, or the removal of the causes. Smoking, dust inhalation and other triggers need to be avoided.
    - As for samshamana treatment to ease bronchitis, many distinct Ayurvedic medications, such as *rasahoushadis* and *kastoushadhi*, are suggested for relieving *kaphaja kasa*.

6. *Kaphaja kasa* is a type of *kasa* dominated by *kapha* and *vata dosha dusti* or imbalance. Ayurveda texts explain the *nidana*, *samprapti* as well as treatment of *kaphaja*

kasa in detail. Chronic bronchitis is a pathological condition characterized by chronic cough and excessive mucous secretion. Thus, Ayurveda plays a major role in its treatment.

7. Ayurveda believes that chronic bronchitis and *kaphaja-kasa* might be connected based on *samprati* (prognosis), *lakshana* (symptoms) and *nidana* (cause). Above all, the *nidana* or causes mentioned by ancient acharyas for the manifestation of *kasa* are: *raja* and *dhuma*, which start the pathological process in *pranavahasamprati* or prognosis of respiratory diseases. Chronic bronchitis appears more commonly in those who smoke regularly and because of frequent dust exposure at work. Treatment for *kaphaja-kasa* involves various forms of *shodhana* (clearance), *nidana parivarjana* (avoiding the causes) and *shamna aushdhi* (*kapha*-decreasing medications). These *shamana* medicines have mucolytic, expectorant and cough suppressant properties.

Key Takeaways:

- Bronchitis (*kasa roga*) in Ayurveda is caused by the imbalance of *vata* and *kapha doshas*, where aggravated *vata* is obstructed by vitiated *kapha*, leading to symptoms like coughing and difficulty breathing. Ayurvedic treatments, including herbal formulations, dietary adjustments, lifestyle changes, pranayama, and yoga, help balance the *doshas* and support the body's natural healing process.
- Bronchitis, or *kasa roga* in Ayurveda, is linked to an imbalance in all three *doshas* – *vata*, *pitta* and *kapha*.

The disease is classified into five types based on *dosha* involvement. The *vata dosha* causes dry cough, *pitta dosha* results in bleeding, fever, and cough, while *kapha dosha* leads to a productive cough. Bronchitis can also arise from injury, infection, or tuberculosis. Ayurvedic treatment emphasizes balancing the *doshas* through herbal remedies, dietary adjustments, and pranayama.

- Ayurveda attributes poor digestion as the main cause of bronchitis, treating it with remedies that support both the digestive system and lungs. Cough (*kasa*) is a sign of *kapha dosha* imbalance, often identified by a coated tongue (*jihva saamta*) and weak gastric fire (*agni*). In chronic bronchitis, known as *kaphaja kasa*, thick sputum and a persistent cough are common symptoms. Ayurveda emphasizes avoiding causative factors, purification therapies (*shodana*), and curative medications (*shamana*) for treatment.
- *Vaman* (therapeutic emesis) and *virechan* (purgation therapy) are effective *panchakarma* treatments for bronchitis. *Vaman* clears excess *kapha* from the respiratory tract, alleviating congestion and mucus. *Virechan* balances *pitta dosha*, speeds metabolism, and aids detoxification. Combined with a tailored diet and lifestyle adjustments, these therapies aim to enhance lung function and reduce bronchitis symptoms.
- Bronchitis shares similarities with *kaphaja kasa* in terms of causative factors like dust, smoke, and diet that aggravate *vata* and *kapha doshas*, along with symptoms such as cough, heavy sputum, difficulty breathing, and dry throat. Managing bronchitis requires halting disease progression through *agnideepana* (enhancing digestive

fire), *amapachana* (detoxification), and *kaphanissarana* (removal of excess mucus). Ancient Ayurvedic texts document these respiratory disorders linked to *kapha* and difficulty breathing.

- *Kaphaja kasa*, dominated by *kapha* and *vata dosha* imbalance, is closely related to chronic bronchitis, which features persistent cough and excessive mucus secretion. Ayurveda provides detailed guidance on the causes, progression, and treatment of *kaphaja kasa*, playing a significant role in managing this condition.

Chapter 11

FUNGAL INFECTIONS

Fungal infections cause circular lesions on the skin which are red, thick and dry; these are frequently clear in the middle, scaly and irritating. They can emerge on any body part that is exposed.

Fungal infections are contagious and can spread from one person to another as well as from one bodily region to another. The most prevalent locations for fungal infections are the underarms, waist, scalp, below the breasts (in females) and inside beard (in males), groin area (jock itch), in the inner part of the thigh and space between the toes (athlete's foot). Fungal infections may include ringworm and candidiasis. Infections caused by fungi typically appear on wet and damp skin.

Signs and Symptoms

- Depending on the location of the infection, there may be a variety of symptoms. Typically, ringworm is the causative factor.
- Circular lesions are occasionally seen; these have vesiculated edges and are itchy, scaly with a clearing in the centre.

According to Ayurveda, fungal infections are caused by an imbalance in the body's *doshas*, which include *vata, pitta* and *kapha*. In particular, an excess of *kapha* and *pitta doshas* is frequently associated with this disease, which causes the body to be overrun by fungi.

Ayurvedic treatment for *dadru* includes local application of *lepa, shamana karma* and *sodhana karma*. It is crucial for the diseased person to expel the vitiated *doshas* by *sodhana chikitsa*. To eliminate the vitiated *pitta* and *rakta*, Ayurveda believes that *dadru kushta virechana* and *raktmokshana* should be administered.

- In a different kind, the ringworm affects the scalp, causing alopecia, itching and scaling, along with dry and brittle hair.
- The groin area, the inner part of the thigh and upper thighs can occasionally become infected with ringworm.
- Scaling, itching and hair loss are some common symptoms of a fungal infection of the scalp. Additionally, as it dries out, the hair becomes brittle.
- Vesicular patches or a well-defined area of intensely irritating and itching pustules may crop up.
- In females, the itching lesions may be present under the breasts, under the arms and in the axillae. In males, ringworm can frequently affect the groin, upper and inner thighs.

Ayurvedic Understanding of the Disease

Generally, when a skin infection is reddish, accompanied by itching, this entails the papules to be of *Dadru* origin. Signs and symptoms of fungal infection bear a resemblance with *dadru kustha.* In most cases, reddish skin infections that itch are indicative of *dadru*-based papules. According to Ayurveda, fungal infection is referred to as *dadru* and an imbalance in the three *doshas* of the body, particularly the *pitta* (fire humour) and *kapha dosha* (phlegm body humour) is the cause. Fungal disease is broadly categorized as a variety of *kshudra kushta.*

Herbs that Help

- *Haldi* or *haridra*
- *Nagarmotha*
- *Jatamansi*
- *Maricha*
- *Tagar*
- *Snuhi*
- *Palash*
- *Madan phala*
- *Karanj patra*
- *Aamaltas patra*
- *Indraju*
- *Guduchi swarasa*
- *Daruharidra*
- *Saptaparni*
- *Atis*
- *Kutaki*
- *Patol*
- *Pittpapda*
- *Chandan*
- *Chakramadh*
- *Kuth*
- *Sarson*
- *Vayavidanga*

- *Pippali*
- *Kustha*
- *Indryan*
- *Murva*
- *Stavari*
- *Anantamul*
- *Tulsi* (holy basil)
- *Triphala* (*Harad, baheda, amla*)
- *Neem or nimb*
- *Vasa*
- *Choti elaychi or ela*
- *Sathpushpa*
- *Chitrak*
- *Harad or haritaki*
- *Patol*
- *Chiryata*
- *Amla*

Recommended Home Remedies

- Apply garlic juice 2–3 times a day to the affected area or areas. The juice can be obtained from pressing or pounding fresh garlic bulbs. Garlic has exceptional anti-infective and anti-fungal qualities.
- Garlic cloves can also be soaked for several hours in mustard oil or olive oil. These cloves may then be crushed and the oil applied on the skin affected by fungal infection.
- Pound radish seeds (*mooli beej*) and mix in a small amount of mustard oil. Apply as *lepa* on the affected skin.

- Make a paste by pounding a piece of fresh, raw turmeric (*haridra*) along with a few *tulsi* or *neem* leaves. Apply this paste twice a day on the affected areas the skin.
- Pound the seeds of the *chakkermard* plant to make a paste, then combine it with radish juice and apply to the afflicted regions.
- Apply *pudina* (mint) juice on the affected skin.
- Make a paste by pounding some fresh *neem* leaves with a little water. Apply the paste on the affected area and leave it on for about 30 minutes.
- As *neem* has strong anti-fungal properties and can help reduce inflammation, apply *neem* oil directly on the infected area twice daily. In case there is more itching, mix *neem* oil in carrier oil, like coconut oil, and then apply it.
- Combine pounded and powdered *neem* leaves with aloe vera gel. Apply this mixture, twice a day, on the infected area. This combination is high in antioxidants, anti-bacterial and anti-fungal properties which work effectively to curb the fungal infection.
- Mix tomato pulp in some coconut oil and locally apply the paste on the affected area using cotton. Wash it off after 30 minutes.
- Turmeric has valuable anti-fungal as well as anti-inflammatory properties. Make a paste bymixing some turmeric powder with water and apply it locally on the affected area.
- Local application of lemongrass oil helps or even bathing daily with a few drops of lemongrass oil added to water is a useful remedy. Lemongrass oil is beneficial for treating fungal infections as it is believed to be high

in anti-oxidants and is particularly useful for treating ringworm. This essential oil also aids stress reduction.

- Mix apple cider vinegar and water in equal proportions and apply the mixture on the infected skin using some cotton. Leave it on for about 30 minutes before washing the area with lukewarm water.
- Mix a few drops of tea tree oil along with a teaspoon of coconut oil. Apply the mixture on the affected skin twice or thrice a day.
- Pound some fresh *tulsi* leaves. Filter the juice through a thin muslin cloth and use it for local application on the site of the fungal infection.
- Add a little coconut oil to camphor (*kapur*). For at least three times a day, apply the same to the affected area.
- Make a paste with a few pounded *neem* leaves and apply it twice or thrice a day on the affected area. Let it dry on your skin. Additionally, mix some freshly ground raw turmeric or turmeric powder and apply.
- Mix *neem* leaf powder with sandalwood water or rose water and make a thick paste. Apply it on the infected area for relief.
- Make a paste out of basil, mint and radish. Add some sesame oil (*til taila*) to it and use it to massage the affected skin.
- In case the fungal infection is in the scalp, massage the scalp with a mixture of coconut oil and camphor. For head bath, add a teaspoon of lemongrass or wheat-grass juice to the water.
- On the surface of the diseased nail, apply some garlic juice. This provides relief from fungal infection.

- Powdered liquorice (*mulethi*) contains anti-fungal, anti-microbial, and anti-inflammatory properties which makes it an essential herb for recovering from fungal infections. For this, mix 2–3 tablespoons of powdered liquorice in half a cup of water and boil for some time. Apply the paste thus formed twice a day on the affected skin for assistance.

Skin conditions are categorized in Ayurvedic medicine under the general title of *kushta*, which is further divided into *maha kushta* and *kshudra kushta*. One of the eighteen varieties of *kushtas* is *dadru kushta*. *Dadru* is a superficial condition that manifests as the *lakshana* or symptoms of *pidaka* (pimples or skin eruptions), *raga* (redness), *kandu* (itching) and *udagata mandala* (raised patches on the skin).

One of the contributing elements of *kushta*, according to Acharya Sushruta, is an unclean lifestyle. It is believed to be primarily caused by the *upsarga* of *krimis* (worms).

Classical Ayurvedic Drugs

- *Khadirarishta*
- *Gandhak rasayana*
- *Shilajit*
- *Sapta siddha lepa*
- *Mahamajak taila*
- *Panch nimbika avleha*
- *Maha bhallatak avleha*
- *Amrit bhallatak avleha*
- *Maha marichyaadi taila*
- *Laghu marichyaadi taila*
- *Kasisaadi ghrit*

- *Bhalatak avleha*
- *Kasmard yoga (lepa)*
- *Moolakbeejaadi yoga (lepa)*
- *Gunjaadi udvartan*
- *Dardaadi lepa*
- *Dadruvidravan malahar*
- *Mayurksharadi lepa*
- *Gunjadh urvartan*
- *Talkodhya malahar*
- *Laghumarichadi taila*
- *Dardadi lepa*
- *Bhalatak avaleha*
- *Kasisadi ghrita*
- *Sarivadya asav*
- *Panchtikt churan*
- *Panchtikt ghrit*
- *Maha manjishthaadi kwath*
- *Laghumanjisthaadi kwath*
- *Kasis badha rasa*
- *Guduchi kwath*
- *Parad bhasma*
- *Mahatikht ghrit*
- *Tikht ghrit*
- *Neel ghrit*
- *Dadru lepa*
- *Vajra shilajit*
- *Maha marichyaadi taila*
- *Kapitth rasa (lepa)*
- *Palash kshar*
- *Guduchi yog*

- *Aaragvadhpatra yog*
- *Manasheela*
- *Paradaadi malham*
- *Ajakarna* (*lepa, snaan, ubatan*)
- *Yograj yog*
- *Kaishor guggulu*
- *Saaribadya asava*
- *Swarna makshika bhasm*
- *Khadira kwatha*
- *Neel ghrita*
- *Triphala*
- *Trikatu*
- *Guduchi ghrita*
- *Triphal ghrita*
- *Nimbadhi ghrita*
- *Kanak bindu aristha*
- *Bhalatak ghrita*
- *Vayavidanga*
- *Kustha-nashak lepa*
- *Masyadhi lepa*
- *Guduchi swaras*
- *Tri yog*
- *Edgajaadi lepa*

Diet and Lifestyle Management Tips

- Keep the affected area clean, hygienic and dry.
- Avoid tight-fitting clothes and wear loose clothes or breathable fabrics.
- Stay hydrated and drink plenty of water to help flush out toxins from the body.

- Eating a healthy and balanced diet high in vitamin C is crucial in addition to the therapy. Follow a diet rich in seasonal fruits, vegetables and whole grains.
- Add more turmeric powder or turmeric milk (*haldi dhoodh*) to your diet.
- Include raw garlic in your diet for its anti-fungal and anti-microbial properties. Garlic also boosts immunity.
- Taking more tomatoes in diet helps as tomatoes contain anti-fungal properties and are a rich source of tartaric acid, succinic acid and citric acid that prevent the growth of fungus spores.
- Practise yoga every day for strength and to get rid of toxins due to fungal infections.
- For this purpose, *kunjal kriya* helps induce vomiting that rids the body of harmful substances, while *shankh prakshalana* acts as a natural purgative.
- Skin ailments can be relieved by performing yoga asanas such as *Sarvangasana, Matsyasana, Pashchimottanasana* and *Surya Namaskar,* as well as yoga techniques like *Jalandhar bandha* and *Uddiyan bandha.*
- As an adjunct to therapy, *pranayama,* or deep breathing exercises, such as *Bhastrika, Kapalbhati, Nadi shodhan* and *Sheetali* may be beneficial.
- If the fungal infection persists, it is essential to consult a healthcare professional or dermatologist prior to stopping any topical anti-fungal creams or drugs and for further evaluation and treatment, if needed.
- Furthermore, as low immunity causes repeated fungal infections, boost your immunity.

Acharya Sushruta states that *dadru kushtha* is a skin condition that manifests as papules, with a copper or bluish colour, and spreads across the skin.

According to Acharya Kashyapa, *dadru* is a skin condition characterized by *vriddhimant mandals* or distributing discoid lesions with severe burning, itching and discharges. The lesions can occasionally be dry in character, which is crucial from a practical standpoint.

As per the reference mentioned in *Agnivesha, Charaka Samhita* and *Shaman Aushadhis* those medicines that can act as *sthanika chikitsa* (static treatment) externally and internally perform *rakta shuddhi* (purification of blood) should be taken in order to cure the disease and to uproot it. The Ayurvedic medications in the form of lepas (local application) work more rapidly due to the physiological consequence of heat on the skin.

Panchakarma

Vaman and *vasti* are two recommended Ayurvedic *panchakarma* treatments for severe fungal infections. *Vaman,* or therapeutic emesis, aids in detoxification by balancing *kapha dosha*, removing toxins and inhibiting the growth of fungi. On the other hand, *vasti*, or medicated enemas, helps get rid of deep-seated impurities, strengthen the immune system and balance the vitiated *vata dosha*. Together, these treatments help to purify the body, balance the *doshic* field and strengthen the skin's natural defence. Certain dietary and lifestyle changes are advised in addition to these therapies to promote general healing and guard against recurrent infections.

Some Ayurvedic facts about Fungal Infections:

1. Fungal infections have a higher incidence and can cause more serious diseases, if left untreated, and

present a significant challenge to clinicians. This ailment is similar to *dadru* kustha in Ayurveda. Scaly, erythematous plaques that are confined and caused by dematophyte infection characterize *dadru* kustha. The presence of utsannamandala (raised circular skin lesions), *kandu* (itching), *raga* (erythyma) and *pidaka* (eruptions) are some of its distinguishing characteristics. It is a form of *kshudra kushta, tridoshaja vyadhi* with dominance of *pitta* and *kapha doshas.* Given its distinctive characteristics, Acharya Charaka classifies *dadru* as a *ksudra kustha*. However, Acharya Sushruta and Vagbhatta classify it as *maha kustha. Pitta* and *kapha dosha* vitiation predominates in this *chirkaalaja* (chronic) *vyadhi.* These Ayurvedic *dadru kustha* symptoms are more typical of fungal infections, which can spread rapidly to other body areas.

2. In *Kashudra Kushtha,* Acharya Charaka described *dadru,* and the majority of Ayurvedic books classify all forms of *kushtha* as *rakta doshaja vikaras* or diseases of the skin. In Ayurveda, *dadru* is one of the *kapha pitta pradhana twak vikaras,* referring to the main causes, or *hetu,* of *dadru* (skin fungal infection), although Acharyas did not explain distinct diagnosis, or *nidana,* for *dadru kushta.* However, it is specified that *malaja krimi* through *sweda* (contact with an infected person's clothing etc.) helps spread *dadru kushta* from person to person. *Dadru* is probably comparable to a fungal skin disease when the fungus spore spreads from a sick individual to a healthy one.
3. The *Kustha Nidana*'s *Brihattrayi* and *Laghutrayi* both refer to the fundamental ideas of *dadru's hetu,* or

causes of the fungal infection. The majority of the *apathya ahara viharas* (unfavourable and incompatible diet and lifestyle measures), listed in Ayurveda as causes of *kushtha*, create a practical environment for the development of fungal infections in skin tissues. According to contemporary science, the clinical signs of *dadru* are quite similar to those of tinea infection, which is brought on by exposure to infectious materials, poor nutrition, stress, obesity and contact with sick people. *Darshana* and *prashana pareeksha* can assess the frequent clinical signs of red spots and severe itching, mentioned in Ayurvedic writings.

4. Skin conditions have been explained well in Ayurveda since Vedic times. Skin, or *tvak*, may be affected by *dadru*, a disease that manifests as *kandu*, mandala and *pidaka*. In this *kapha-pitta pradhana* disease, the symptoms are very similar to those of tinea or fungal infection.

    - Ayurvedic classics define fungal diseases as *dadru* and *sidhma*, which fall under the kustha category. *Dadru* is comparable to other types of fungal illnesses, while *sidhma* is likened to *yinea* versicolor. *Darshana* and *prashana pariksha* can diagnose the common clinical symptoms of red patches and excessive, intense itching.

5. *Dadru* equates to a *shabdha*, or word, which translates to tortoise, according to an old scripture called *Shabda Kalpa Druma*. This is because *dadru* falls under *anadaya shabda roopa*, which indicates that it lacks any *dhatu* or *pratyaya*.

- *Dadru* is consequently thought to be a form of leprosy (*kushta*, or skin disease) that is characterized by tortoise-like skin sores.
- *Dadru rogino naama, saa asyaastiti dadrunaha, dadruna ithi-deeryanteanya charma daruhu.*
- *Dadru rogi* is a person who has skin lesions that cause the continuous loss of normal skin, or one who suffers from *dadru* (*manushya varga, amarakosha dwiteeya*).
- *Dadru* is described as a kind of *kshudra kushta* with tortoise-like traits in Vaidyaka Shabda Sindhu.

6. In modern medicine, fungal infection, that is tinea/ ringworm, is correlated to *dadru kushta* due to similarities in their symptoms.
   - Ayurveda skin infection is termed as *twak vikara* or *kushta roga*. *Dadru* is one of the *kushta rogas* and termed as a *dadru kushta*. According to most of Ayurveda texts, all types of *kushta* are considered as *rakta doshaja vikara*. *Dadru* is one of the *kapha-pitta pradhana twak vikara*.

Key Takeaways:

- Ayurveda attributes fungal infections, like *dadru*, to imbalances in *vata*, *pitta*, and *kapha doshas*, particularly an excess of *kapha* and *pitta*. Treatment involves local applications (*lepa*), and both *shamana* (palliative) and *sodhana* (purification) therapies. To eliminate vitiated *pitta* and *rakta*, *virechana* (purgation) and *raktmokshana* (bloodletting) are recommended to restore balance.

- In Ayurveda, skin infections that are reddish and itchy are often associated with *dadru*, a type of fungal infection. This condition is believed to arise from an imbalance in the body's *doshas*, primarily the *pitta* (fire) and *kapha* (phlegm). Fungal infections like *dadru* are categorized under *kshudra kushta*, a general term for minor skin diseases. Treatment focuses on balancing the *doshas* through purification and local therapies.
- In Ayurvedic medicine, skin conditions are broadly classified as *kushta*, which is further subdivided into maha *kushta* (major) and *kshudra kushta* (minor). *Dadru kushta*, one of the eighteen types of *kushta*, is a superficial skin condition characterized by symptoms such as pimples or skin eruptions (*pidaka*), redness (*raga*), itching (*kandu*), and raised patches (*udagata mandala*). According to Acharya Sushruta, poor lifestyle and an imbalance caused by *krimis* (worms) are key contributing factors to *kushta*, especially *dadru*.
- *Vaman* and *vasti* are effective *panchakarma* treatments for severe fungal infections. *Vaman*, or therapeutic emesis, helps in detoxification by balancing *kapha dosha*, clearing toxins, and preventing fungal growth. *Vasti*, or medicated enemas, targets deep-seated impurities, strengthens the immune system, and balances *vata dosha*. Together, these therapies purify the body, restore *dosha* balance, and enhance the skin's natural defenses. Additionally, Ayurvedic dietary and lifestyle adjustments are recommended to promote healing and prevent recurring infections.
- *Dadru*, a type of skin fungal infection, is classified under *kapha-pitta* skin disorders in Ayurveda. It is

spread through contact with infected materials, such as clothing, and is linked to malaja *krimi* (worms). While distinct diagnosis for *dadru* is not specified, it is considered a *rakta doshaja vikaras* (disease of the skin).

- *Dadru* is an Ayurvedic term for fungal skin diseases, similar to tinea, and falls under the kustha category. It is characterized by red patches and intense itching, with diagnosis based on clinical symptoms like *kandu*, *mandala*, and *pidaka*.

Chapter 12

SCIATICA

Sciatica or *Sciatic Neuritis* is a painful condition of sciatic nerve neuralgia or painful nerve condition experienced in the buttock region, back of the thigh and in the leg area. It is generally characterized by pain that exudes along the path of the sciatic nerve. An x-ray of the lower back may be required for diagnosis and severity assessment.

Signs and Symptoms

- A sensation of pain travels along the region of the sciatic nerve. It starts from the buttock and radiates down in the posterior aspect of the thigh and calf region, and in the outer border of the foot.
- The pain mainly emits from the lumbar spine to the buttocks and then goes down the back of the leg. This may be in the form of a mild ache or a sharp, burning sensation or severe piercing pain. The pain worsens due to sitting, standing or with forceful movements for a long time.

- Numbness and tingling sensation may be felt in the region of the concerned nerve.
- The affected leg is weak, which also impairs activities such as walking, standing or even lifting the leg.
- Often, movement becomes restricted while lifting the leg.
- Also, reflexes in the affected leg region are reduced, which results in an abnormal posture or gait so as to minimize the pain being experienced.

Ayurvedic Understanding of the Disease

Sciatica, or *gridhrasi* in Ayurveda, is believed to be caused due to the vitiation of the *vata* and *kapha doshas* or the air and phlegm body humours. It is also probable that chronic and long-term constipation may aggravate the disease.

In *gridhrasi*, pain radiates from the lower back to the legs. The term *gridhrasi* is derived from the word *gridhra*, which means a vulture, thus reflecting the limping gait of a vulture. This pain comes with a great deal of inflexibility and lack of sensation, along with a feeling of pins and needles in the affected areas of the lower back, buttocks and the legs. As the disease progresses, there may be weakness in the muscles of the leg or foot and trouble in walking.

Herbs that Help

- *Ashwagandha* (Withania somnifera)
- *Haldi* (Curcuma longa)
- *Guggul* (Commiphora mukul)
- *Nirgundi* (Vitex negundo)
- *Shallaki* (Boswellia serrata)
- *Bala* (Sida cordifolia)

- *Adrak* (Gingiber officinales)
- *Rasna* (Pluchea lanceolata)
- *Eranda* (Ricinus communis)
- *Dashamool* (Ten roots)

Recommended Home Remedies

- Crush 2–4 cloves of garlic and take it with a glassful of warm water early in the morning.
- You can dry a few leaves of the herb *harsingar* or *parijat* (Nyctanthes arbour-tristis) in shade and pound it into a powder. Mix about 3 grams of this herb powder with honey and take twice a day.
- Take *hing* (asafoetida) in the dosage of approx. 125–500mg.
- Mix a few strands of saffron in half to one cup of warm to hot milk and drink it at bedtime.
- Mix 1–3 grams of turmeric powder in a glass of milk and add a pinch of black pepper to the same to increase absorption. Boil the mixture and drink it hot once or twice a day.
- You may take some crude castor oil, at bedtime, in a dose of 1–2 teaspoons, mixed in milk.
- Soak half a teaspoon of *methi dana* (fenugreek seeds). Chew themon empty stomach in the morning. Also, drink the water used for soaking the seeds.
- Drink ginger tea 2–3 times a day to aid the reduction of inflammation and pain.
- Mix 1 gram each of dried ginger powder (*saunth*) and *pippali* powder in 5–10 ml of castor oil. Take this mixture once or twice daily for a few days.
- Massage the painful area with warm cove oil.

Classical Ayurvedic Drugs

- *Yograj guggul*
- *Maha yograj guggul*
- *Maha narayan taila* (local massage)
- *Trayodashang guggul*
- *Bala taila* (local massage)
- *Sameer pannag rasa*
- *Kubaj prasarini taila* (local massage)
- *Maharasnadi kwath*
- *Sihnad guggul*
- *Jeerakadyarisht*
- *Maha rasnaadi guggul*
- *Dashamoola kashaya*
- *Vat kulantak ras*
- *Brihat vat chintamani ras*
- *Sameer gaja kesari*
- *Rasnasaptak kwath*
- *Balarishta*
- *Vaishvanar churan*
- *Erand taila* (local massage)
- *Maha vishgarbh taila* (local massage)
- *Saindhavaadi taila* (local massage)
- *Vishamushti vati*
- *Ashwagandharisht*
- *Dashmool ghrit*
- *Erand pak*
- *Tambulaadi churan*
- *Dashmoolarisht*
- *Nirgundi taila* (local massage)
- *Rasnaerandadi kashayam*

Classical Ayurvedic works like *agnikarma, panchakarma* and *siravedha,* along with *nidana, samprapti, lakshana* and *chikitsa* are suggested for the management of sciatica or *gridhrasi*.

In *gridhrasi*, *bhava misra* also supports *chikitsa vamana,* which Chakrapani indicates is practised following *snehana* and *svedana* activities. Moreover, it is mentioned that *vamana* does not play a role in the *vataja* kind of *gridhrasi*, but it would be useful in the *vata-kaphaja type.*

In the case of *gridhrasi*, *virechana* or the purgation therapy also plays a significant part. Mild *virechana* is enough in *gridhrasi* as it helps to bring out the vitiated *doshas* from *amashaya* and *pakvashaya* (stomach and intestines).

Diet and Lifestyle Management Tips

Managing sciatica through diet and lifestyle changes can be considerably helpful in reducing its symptoms and preventing recurrence of the disease. In addition, constipation, indigestion and flatulence should be corrected initially to control the disease.

- Add more garlic and turmeric to meals.
- It is good to drink herbal tea made using *nirgundi* and/ or *rasna* would be good.
- Minimise the consumption of uncooked, cold and dried food as they tend to cause *vata dosha* aggravation.
- Consume warm and freshly cooked foods, as well as nutritious, whole grains warming oils like sesame seed oil or mustard oil and ghee, which are light to digest. These help to alleviate and pacify the *dosha* vitiation and particularly assist in reducing *vata dosha* imbalance.

- Add warming spices and condiments like cumin, fennel, turmeric, and black pepper to everyday diet options to aid digestion and reduce inflammation.
- It also helps to eat seasonal and cooked vegetables, as well as seasonal fruits, possibly cooked or stewed.
- Avoid fast foods, processed foods and carbonated drinks that tend to aggravate *vata dosha*.
- Drink warm to hot water throughout the day.
- Hot fomentation with a bag of salt or sand is advised.
- Wear warm and comfortable clothes, especially around the leg area and the lower back. This helps to protect the area from external cold and dampness.
- Tak warm water baths and use warm compresses or heating pads on the affected area to reduce stiffness and pain.
- Practise mild and comfortable exercises like yoga (along with stretching asanas/yoga poses of *Pawanmuktasana, Bhujangasana* and *Shalabhasana*), walking in fresh air and swimming in warm water. These improve flexibility and strengthen the leg muscles.
- Gently massage the affected leg with warm castor oil and leave it on for a few hours for relief.
- A proper and good posture is needed while sitting, standing, as well as during sleeping to reduce the strain on the lower back and the leg.
- Relaxing and rejuvenating routines and activities help as these aid in stress management.
- Optimum sleeping and adequate rest are required, along with avoiding overexertion in any form.

Gridhrasi is a type of neuralgic disease which affects the muscles supplied by the sciatic nerve. Due to its direct connection to the locomotor system, this condition causes the person a significant deal of distress and interferes with daily activities.

It is recommended to use *vedanasthapana chikitsa* (analgesic), *shothahara* (anti-inflammatory) and *vata dosha nivarana* (*vata* pacifying treatment). The Ayurvedic management for *sciatica* comprises both *shodhana* (internal cleansing) and *shamana* (oral medication) therapies.

Panchakarma

Vasti and *kati vasti* are the main *panchakarma* treatments in Ayurveda for sciatica. By balancing the *vata dosha, vasti* (medicated enemas) reduces inflammation and pain, along with the associated of sciatica. *Kati vasti* is a localized treatment by the application of warm medicinal oil on the lower back to relieve pain and stiffness. These treatments are meant to improve range of motion, reduce discomfort and encourage recovery. When paired with particular food and lifestyle suggestions, these therapies offer all-encompassing alleviation of the disease symptoms and promote general spinal health.

Some Ayurvedic facts about Sciatica:

1. *Gridhrasi* (sciatica) is regarded as one of the major *vata vyadhi* (neurological diseases) in Ayurveda.

    - *Gridhrasi* types mentioned in Ayurveda are: *vataja gridhrasi* and *vata kaphaja gridhrasi.* Although, there is little or no explanation of the *purvarupa* (initial signs) of *gridhrasi* in the classics, yet,

Charaka claims the avyakta *lakshana* (unidentified symptoms) to be the *purvarupas* (initial symptoms) of the *vata vyadhi*, while *gridhrasi* is identified as a *vata vyadhi*.

- *Gridhrasi* rupa, or the signs and symptoms of sciatica, are characterized by *ruk* (pain), *toda* (pricking sensation), *muhu spandana* (tingling sensation) and *stambha* (stiffness). In case of *vataja gridhrasi*, this includes feeling pain in the foot, calf, knee, hip and the back of the thigh.

2. The word *gridhrasi* is derived from the Sanskrit word gridhra, or vulture. This is so because the patient suffering from this disease walks like a vulture. In other words, there is a typical gait associated with a sciatica patient – slightly tilted at the affected side with the affected leg in a flexed position and the other leg extended.

    - From the period of Maharishi Charaka and Sushruta, this disease has been described in classical texts by the name of *gridhrasi* and has been included in the eighty types of *nanatmaja vatavyadhi*, or diseases in which the *vata dosha* becomes aggravated and vitiated.

3. According to Ayurvedic perception, sciatica is comparable to *gridhrasi*, which is a *nanatmaja vataja vikara*. According to Ayurveda, one of the most common *vata* disorders is *gridhrasi*, which is analogous to sciatica in terms of the patient's stride that shows a vulture-like

appearance due to the individual's severe, continuous and radiating agony.

- For the sciatica disease and for neuropathy, Ayurveda states that *haridra*, or turmeric, is an efficient remedy. This is because it contains curcumin, a potent antioxidant with analgesic and anti-inflammatory effects, which help to reduce the chronic pain and also alleviate the tingling sensation and numbness associated with peripheral neuropathy in the affected region.

4. The four main symptoms of *gridhrasi* (*vataja vikara*), i.e. a *vata dosha* disease, are *ruk* (pain), *toda* (pricking sensation), *muhu spandana* (tingling sensation) and *stambha* (stiffness). There may also be *aruchi* (anorexia), *gaurava* (heaviness) and *tandra* (drowsiness) in *vata-kaphaja gridhrasi*. The Ayurvedic treatments for *gridhrasi* (sciatica) are *agnikarma*, *siravedhya* and *bastikarma*.

- As for relieving the disease, *shamana chikitsa*, *patrapinda swedana*, *kati basti*, and *sarvanga abhyanga swedana* procedures have been mentioned.
- Additionally, Charaka asserts that abhyanga is advantageous for the *vata vyadhi* as *vayu* dominates *sparsha indriya* or the sensation of touch.
- Acharya Shushruta has also recommended *sarvanga abhyanga*, or full body massage, with *nirgundi taila* and *murivenna* for *vata shamaka*, or reducing *vata dosha* aggravation.

5. Following a review of the classics, the following are the treatments for *Gridhrasi*:

- ***Snehana***: In the disease of *gridhrasi*, *snehana*, or oleation therapy, is recommended, both for internal as well as external use. Externally, *snehana* might take the shape of *pariseka*, *avagaha*, *abhyanga*, etc. Internally, *snehapana* would be *shamana* and *shodhana* therapy for *mridu roga*, or the milder form of the disease, as mentioned in Ayurvedic literature.
- ***Svedana***: Ayurveda classics mention a great number of svedas, or steam therapy, but not all of them are useful or feasible in *gridhrasi*. *Avagaha* and *pinda svedana* are two types of *svedas* suggested for sciatica or *gridhrasi*. These include pinda sveda and *baluka sveda*, also known as *ruksha sveda*.

  Gridhrasi comes under *nanatamja vata vyadhi*, in which the lower limbs and the back experience extreme pain. *Gridhrasi* can be correlated to sciatica because of similar clinical presentation.

  - The Ayurvedic treatment for sciatica includes both *shodhana* (cleansing or purification therapies) and *shamana* (oral medicine), using *vedanasthapana chikitsa* (analgesics), *shothahara* (anti-inflammatory) and *vata dosha* pacifying treatments.
  - *Gridhrasi* causes great discomfort to the patient and affects his/her everyday practices as it is directly related to the locomotor system.

- *Gridhrasi* falls under the category of *nanatamja vata vyadhi*. In addition to *stambha* (stiffness), *toda* (pricking pain) and *spandana* (twitching), the symptoms of *gridhrasi* include *ruk* (pain), which originates in *sphik* (buttock region) and spreads to *kati* (lower back), *prishtha* (back), *uru* (thigh), *janu* (knee), *jangha* (calf) and *pada* (foot). This is accompanied by *shakti kshepa nigraha*, or the inability to raise the lower limbs.

- There are two types of sciatica based on *dosha* involvement: *vataja* and *vata-kaphaja*.
- If *kapha* is linked to *vata*, then *gridhrasi* may also exhibit *tandra* (drowsiness), *gaurava* (heaviness) and *arochaka* (anorexia).

- *Gridhrasi* is caused by an aggravated *vata dosha* that invades the *kandras* of the ankles and toes, causing *kshepa* in the thigh region, i.e. pain and inability to extend.

    - Acharya Charaka describes *Gridhrasi* in the *Charaka Samhita*. Beginning at the hip region, the disease of *Gridhrasi* progressively spreads to the waist, back, thigh, knee, shank and foot, causing stiffness, discomfort and piercing pain, in addition to regular shaking. *Gridhrasi* corresponds to the disease of sciatica, which is a painful health condition that begins in the lumbar area and extends to the leg and the posterior-lateral aspect of the thighs. Sciatica is a common *vata vyadhi* and requires a multimodal strategy to manage pain, disability and other issues.

KEY TAKEAWAYS:

- Sciatica, or *gridhrasi*, in Ayurveda is caused by vitiated *vata* and *kapha doshas*, with chronic constipation potentially aggravating it. The pain radiates from the lower back to the legs, accompanied by inflexibility, numbness, and tingling sensations. The condition can also lead to muscle weakness and difficulty walking as it progresses.
- For managing sciatica (*gridhrasi*), Ayurvedic treatments like *agnikarma*, *panchakarma*, and *siravedha* are recommended, along with assessing *nidana*, *samprapti*, *lakshana*, and *chikitsa*. *Vamana* therapy is useful in *vata-kaphaja gridhrasi*, after *snehana* and *svedana*, but not in *vataja* types. *Virechana*, or purgation, also plays a key role, with mild purgation helping to eliminate vitiated *doshas* from the stomach and intestines.
- *Gridhrasi*, or sciatica, is a neuralgic condition that affects muscles supplied by the sciatic nerve, causing significant distress and disrupting daily activities. Ayurvedic management includes *vedanasthapana chikitsa* (analgesic), *shothahara* (anti-inflammatory), and *vata dosha nivarana* (*vata* pacifying treatment). Both *shodhana* (internal cleansing) and *shamana* (oral medication) therapies are used for effective treatment.
- *Vasti* and *kati vasti* are key Ayurvedic treatments for sciatica, balancing *vata dosha*, reducing pain and inflammation, and improving mobility. These therapies, combined with specific food and lifestyle recommendations, help alleviate symptoms and promote spinal health.

- *Gridhrasi*, or sciatica, is named after the vulture due to the typical limping gait it causes. Described in classical texts by Charaka and Sushruta, it is part of the eighty types of *vata*-related diseases.
- The main symptoms of *gridhrasi* (sciatica) include pain, pricking sensation, tingling, and stiffness. Additional symptoms may include anorexia, heaviness, and drowsiness in *vata-kaphaja* cases. Ayurvedic treatments include *agnikarma*, *siravedhya* and *bastikarma*.

INDEX

Acknowledgements

I am highly grateful to the Almighty who has once again given me this splendid opportunity to write another book and connect with one and all, rendering proficient connectivity of our innate Science of Ayurveda with providing healing solutions for solemn ailments. And definitely I do acknowledge the contributions of Ayurvedic scholars, researches and practitioners who have set norms of substantial study and practice of Ayurveda. It has certainly inspired me and as well informed my work as writer and author. And heartfelt thanks to my loving family, to have always supported me and guided on my endeavour to reach out to masses with the efficient Ayurvedic healthcare remedies.

